ICD-11 Personality Disorders

About the Authors

Bo Bach, PhD, DMSc, is clinical professor at Copenhagen University Hospital in Slagelse, where he works as clinician and director of the Center for Personality Disorder Research. Bach was granted the 2021 Theodore Millon Award by the American Psychological Association for his mid-career contribution to the assessment of Personality Disorders. He is co-author of the *Diagnostic Interview for Personality Pathology in ICD-11* (DIPP-11) and the *Personality Disorder Severity for ICD-11* (PDS-ICD-11) scale. He served as a consultant for WHO on the development of the ICD-11 classification of Personality Disorders and associated field trials. He is a former board member of the European Society for the Study of Personality Disorders (ESSPD) and serves on the editorial board for *Personality Disorders: Theory, Research, and Treatment* and *Journal of Personality Assessment*. Bach is an internationally certified trainer and supervisor in schema therapy.

Sebastian Simonsen, PhD, is scientific director and clinical practitioner at Stolpegaard Psychotherapy Centre, Mental Health Services in Copenhagen. He is also an affiliated associate professor at the University of Copenhagen. As a scientist–practitioner, Simonsen is specialized in Personality Disorders with a particular focus on clinical management, treatment planning, psychotherapy, psychopathology, mentalization, social cognition, and interpersonal avoidance. He was part of the work group behind the Danish national guidelines for borderline personality disorder and has published a review paper on European guidelines. Internationally, he has contributed to the dissemination of new dimensional models of Personality Disorders as well as mentalization-based therapy (MBT). He is also a former board member of the European Society for the Study of Personality Disorders (ESSPD) and serves on the editorial board for *Journal of Clinical Psychology*. Simonsen is an internationally certified trainer and supervisor in MBT.

ICD-11 Personality Disorders

A Clinician's Guide

Bo Bach and Sebastian Simonsen

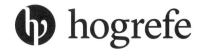

Library of Congress of Congress Cataloging in Publication information for the print version of this book is available via the Library of Congress Marc Database under the Library of Congress Control Number 2024948423

Library and Archives Canada Cataloguing in Publication

Title: ICD-11 personality disorders : a clinician's guide / Bo Bach and Sebastian Simonsen.

Other titles: ICD-11 personlighedsforstyrrelser. English

Names: Bach, Bo, author. | Simonsen, Sebastian, author.

Description: Translation of: ICD-11 personlighedsforstyrrelser: en klinisk vejledning. | Includes bibliographical references. | In English, translated from the Danish.

Identifiers: Canadiana (print) 2024048746X | Canadiana (ebook) 20240487575 | ISBN 9780889376489 (softcover) | ISBN 9781616766481 (PDF) | ISBN 9781613346488 (EPUB)

Subjects: LCSH: Personality disorders. | LCSH: Personality disorders—Diagnosis. | LCSH: Personality disorders—Treatment.

Classification: LCC RC554 .B3313 2024 | DDC 616.85/81—dc23

Original title: *ICD-11 Personlighedsforstyrrelser – En Klinisk Vejledning* by Bo Bach and Sebastian Simonsen. (ISBN 978-87-7135-112-5), published under license from Hogrefe Psykologisk Forlag, A/S, Denmark.

© 2023 by Hogrefe Psykologisk Forlag A/S

© 2025 by Hogrefe Publishing

www.hogrefe.com

The authors and publisher have made every effort to ensure that the information contained in this text is in accord with the current state of scientific knowledge, recommendations, and practice at the time of publication. In spite of this diligence, errors cannot be completely excluded. Also, due to changing regulations and continuing research, information may become outdated at any point. The authors and publisher disclaim any responsibility for any consequences which may follow from the use of information presented in this book.

Registered trademarks are not noted specifically as such in this publication. The use of descriptive names, registered names, and trademarks does not imply, even in the absence of a specific statement, that such names are exempt from the relevant protective laws and regulations and therefore free for general use.

The cover image is an agency photo depicting models. Use of the photo on this publication does not imply any connection between the content of this publication and any person depicted in the cover image.
Cover image: © gremlin - iStock.com

PUBLISHING OFFICES

USA: Hogrefe Publishing Corporation, 44 Merrimac St., Newburyport, MA 01950
            Phone 978 255 3700; E-mail customersupport@hogrefe.com

EUROPE: Hogrefe Publishing GmbH, Merkelstr. 3, 37085 Göttingen, Germany
            Phone +49 551 99950 0, Fax +49 551 99950 111; E-mail publishing@hogrefe.com

SALES & DISTRIBUTION

USA: Hogrefe Publishing, Customer Services Department,
            30 Amberwood Parkway, Ashland, OH 44805
            Phone 800 228 3749, Fax 419 281 6883; E-mail customersupport@hogrefe.com

EUROPE: Hogrefe Publishing, Merkelstr. 3, 37085 Göttingen, Germany
            Phone +49 551 99950 0, Fax +49 551 99950 111; E-mail publishing@hogrefe.com

OTHER OFFICES

CANADA: Hogrefe Publishing Corporation, 82 Laird Drive, East York, Ontario, M4G 3V1

SWITZERLAND: Hogrefe Publishing, Länggass-Strasse 76, 3012 Bern

Printed and bound in the Czech Republic

ISBN 978-0-88937-648-9 (print) · ISBN 978-1-61676-648-1 (PDF) · ISBN 978-1-61334-648-8 (EPUB)
https://doi.org/10.1027/00648-000

Preface

It has long been anticipated that the World Health Organization's (2024) *International Statistical Classification of Diseases* (11th ed.; ICD-11) would introduce a fundamentally new dimensional classification of Personality Disorders, which eventually turned out to become a lengthy process characterised by controversies and postponements. It is never easy for humankind to agree on and adapt to new frameworks and procedures. So, it was hardly believable when the new ICD-11 approach was officially launched in 2022 for translation and implementation in World Health Organization member countries.

Due to the aforementioned circumstances, we are convinced that the transition to the ICD-11 classification of Personality Disorders requires comprehensive preparation and retraining in clinical settings. Thus, we have decided to write this introductory book aimed at clinical practitioners as well as interested students and scholars.

The process of writing this book has certainly benefited from our collaboration with people such as Michael B. First, Geoffrey M. Reed, W. John Livesley, Christopher J. Hopwood, Jared W. Keeley, Robert F. Krueger, Anthony Bateman, Joost Hutsebaut, Giancarlo Dimaggio, Lois W. Choi-Kain, Donna S. Bender, Peter Tyrer, Carla Sharp, Steven K. Huprich, Lee Anna Clark, and, last but definitely not least, Martin Sellbom and Roger Mulder.

We also extend our gratitude to the European Society of the Study of Personality Disorders, the International Society for the Study of Personality Disorders, the British and Irish Group for the Study of Personality Disorders, and the Royal College of Psychiatrists for organising debates, workshops, and lectures on the ICD-11 classification of Personality Disorders. We particularly thank Sabine Herpertz, Giles Newton-Howes, Oliver Dale, Andrew M. Chanen, Babette Renneberg, Tennyson Lee, Ueli Kramer, and Michaela Swales.

We also owe great thanks to our local Scandinavian collaborators, in particular Erik Simonsen who originally paved the way for our careers in the field of Personality Disorder research and clinical practice. Along these lines, we would like to acknowledge our professional home bases under the auspices of the Slagelse Psychiatric Hospital, Region Zealand; Stolpegaard Psychotherapy Centre in Gentofte, Capital Region; and the Institute for Personality Theory and Psychopathology.

And last, we would like to thank our editors Lisa Bennett and Christian Aarestrup at Hogrefe for a very pleasant and helpful process of preparing this book.

Bo Bach and Sebastian Simonsen, August 2024

Contents

Chapter 1

Background

With the introduction of the World Health Organization's (2024) *Clinical Descriptions and Diagnostic Requirements for ICD-11 Mental, Behavioural and Neurodevelopmental Disorders* there has been a paradigm shift in the way we understand and diagnose Personality Disorder. In this introductory chapter, we will describe the most important changes and their underlying clinical and scientific rationale as a starting point for the remaining chapters of the book.

The Purpose of This Book

ICD-11's classification of Personality Disorder can be said to contain significant changes that require fundamental retraining of professionals as well as restructuring of clinical practice in general. In an attempt to support this challenging process, we have chosen to write a book that we hope clinicians will find useful for this purpose. We recommend that readers use the book as a guide that can be consulted as needed and should not necessarily be read from start to finish. For example, clinicians may want to begin by reading the section "A Crash Course in the Clinical Use of Personality Functioning and Traits" in Chapter 2 to understand the clinical rationale for the new classification. Chapter 2 also includes extensive differential diagnostic guidelines, which may be helpful in clinical practice. Next, it can be beneficial to familiarise yourself with the different capacities and manifestations of personality functioning in Chapter 3, which form the basis for the crucial assessment and description of severity in Chapter 4. Furthermore, Chapter 5 can be used to gain an overview of the five trait domains that describe the style and expression of the patient's personality disturbances. When considering treatment options, it may be helpful to consult Chapter 6 for specific suggestions described for each level of severity as well as different combinations of trait domains. In the book's appendix, we have chosen to include extra features that may be useful ("nice to know") but not absolutely necessary ("need to know") to get started using the new classification.

As a general clarification for readers, we tend to use terms such as "personality dysfunction," "personality difficulties," and "personality disturbances" interchangeably. These terms are not diagnostic entities as such but apply to human personality functioning in a broader sense. The official ICD-11 classification is explicitly and exclusively referred to in terms of "Personality Difficulty," "Mild Personality Disorder," "Moderate Personality Disorder," and "Severe Personality Disorder" along with the five trait domain specifiers (i.e., Negative Affectivity, Detachment, Dissociality, Disinhibition, and Anankastia) and the Borderline pattern specifier.

Brief Introduction to ICD-11 Personality Disorder

With ICD-11, Personality Disorder is described and diagnosed based on what it actually means to be a person, psychologically speaking, and in particular what it means to struggle with personality issues (Bender, 2019; Sharp & Wall, 2021; Tyrer et al., 2019). In short, ICD-11 guides us to diagnose Personality Difficulty and Personality Disorder based on general impairments in aspects of the self and interpersonal functioning, along with emotional, cognitive, and behavioural manifestations, as well as global psychosocial functioning and distress. Once these general aspects of personality functioning and manifestations are found to be present in the patient, the diagnosis can be further classified by severity (i.e., mild, moderate, severe) or the sub-diagnostic presence of Personality Difficulty. This can be further supplemented with a specification of one or more of the most prominent trait domains (i.e., Negative Affectivity, Detachment, Dissociality, Disinhibition, and Anankastia) in order to emphasise the individual expression of the diagnosis. Finally, there is also the option to further specify a code for a Borderline pattern when this can make a difference to the patient's treatment. As shown in Table 1.1, only the first cluster of ICD-11 codes, that is, up to and including the severity levels, are generally used as the actual diagnoses, while the trait domains and Borderline pattern are only used as informative additional codes. With the World Health Organization's (1992) *International Statistical Classification of Diseases* (10th ed.; ICD-10), clinicians applied 10 different types of Personality Disorder diagnoses, which in practice are completely equal in terms of severity. It is well known that several Personality Disorder types usually apply to the same patient (i.e., co-occurrence). With ICD-11, the focus has instead shifted to categories of overall severity, while the style or typology can be described using trait domains (see examples in Appendix B). For a more concrete introduction, we refer to the section "Crash Course in the Clinical Use of Personality Functioning and Traits" in Chapter 2.

Table 1.1   Classification of Personality Disorder in ICD-10 and ICD-11

ICD-10	ICD-11
Categories	**Personality Disorder**
60.0 Paranoid	10.Z Severity Unspecified
60.1 Schizoid	**Level of severity**
60.2 Dissocial	50.7 Personality Difficulty
60.3 Emotionally Unstable	(Sub-diagnostic)
[Borderline]	10.0 *Mild* Personality Disorder
60.4 Histrionic	10.1 *Moderate* Personality Disorder
60.5 Anankastic	10.2 *Severe* Personality Disorder
60.6 Anxious [Avoidant]	**Additional specifier codes**
60.7 Dependent	11.0 Negative Affectivity
60.8 Other Specific Type	11.1 Detachment
60.9 Unspecified	11.2 Dissociality
61.0 Mixed Type	11.3 Disinhibition
Z73.1 Accentuation of Personality	11.4 Anankastia
Traits (Sub-diagnostic)	11.5 Borderline pattern

The Creation of a New Classification

The now official ICD-11 classification of Personality Disorder was created through a lengthy and difficult process led by an international working group appointed by the World Health Organization (WHO). The working group was broadly constituted to ensure diverse expertise and geographical representation (Tyrer, 2005; Tyrer et al., 2019; Tyrer, Crawford, & Mulder, 2011). The original working group included Peter Tyrer (psychiatrist) from the UK, Mike Crawford (psychiatrist) from the UK, Roger Mulder (psychiatrist) from New Zealand, Roger Blashfield (psychologist) from the USA, Alireza Farnam (psychiatrist) from Iran, Andrea Fossati (psychologist) from Italy, Michaela Swales (psychologist) from Wales, Dusica Lecic-Tosevski (psychiatrist) from Serbia, David Ndetei (psychiatrist) from Kenya, Nestor Koldobsky (psychiatrist) from Argentina, and Lee Anna Clark (psychologist) from the USA.

Since its launch over 30 years ago, the ICD-10 ("blue book") has explicitly recognised the scientific and practical problems with the classification of Personality Disorder and pointed out a need for a new classification: "a new approach to the description of Personality Disorders is required" (World Health Organization, 1992, p. 20). At the same time, there has been broad agreement in the literature about these problems, while there has been less agreement about how to specifically address them (Clark, 2007; Ekselius et al., 1993; Frances, 1980; Kiesler, 1986; Skodol et al., 2013; Tyrer & Alexander, 1979; Tyrer & Johnson, 1996; Widiger & Trull, 2007).

This is where the WHO ICD-11 working group comes in. Based on a review of the literature, the working group concluded that the core of Personality Disorders lies in basic personality functioning, which can range from healthy functioning to severe dysfunction (Crawford et al., 2011). Based on this initial model, Personality Disorder was mainly defined as the degree of interpersonal dysfunction, that is, the impact on social roles and occupational functions, the "contact" with the patient, and interpersonal risk behaviours (Tyrer, Crawford, Mulder et al., 2011). In addition, stylistic characteristics could be specified using five trait domains that are broadly compatible with the "Big Five" (Mulder et al., 2011; Widiger & Simonsen, 2005). The first proposal for Personality Disorder in ICD-11 was commented on by several international researchers and clinical experts (Davidson, 2011). Several expressed concern about the loss of important knowledge within the traditional categories of Personality Disorder, particularly the diagnosis of Borderline Personality Disorder, while others pointed out problems with moving to a system without a priori evidence of increased clinical utility (Bateman, 2011). In addition to discussions in journals and at conferences, WHO also sought feedback from international members of the World Psychiatric Association and the International Union of Psychological Science. In parallel, the pillars of the draft in question were examined in a number of studies (Kim et al., 2014, 2015, 2016; Mulder et al., 2016; Tyrer et al., 2014).

But the concerns and objections continued. In December 2016, representatives from the European Society for the Study of Personality Disorders wrote a letter addressed to the person responsible for the chapter on mental disorders in ICD-11, Geoffrey M. Reed. In the letter, the society expressed concern about the current proposal and requested that it be rejected by WHO. A rewritten version of the letter was later published by a number of researchers and clinical experts associated with the European Society for the Study of Personality Disorders, the North American Society for the Study of Personality Disorders, and the International Society for the Study of Personality Disorders (Herpertz et al., 2017). A significant part of the problem was the fact that the previous proposal completely excluded the borderline diagnosis from the classification, as well as concerns that the new model could lead to a loss of valuable knowledge rooted in the traditional categories. Among other things, it was argued that patients with a borderline diagnosis could risk not receiving evidence-based care and lose goodwill if their diagnosis was no longer included in the classification. Based on subsequent meetings in Heidelberg in 2017 with representatives from the WHO working group and representatives from the International Society for the

Study of Personality Disorders, the European Society for the Study of Personality Disorders, and the North American Society for the Study of Personality Disorders, it was decided to adjust the ICD-11 classification to address significant aspects of the criticism. First and foremost, the option to code a Borderline pattern was added as an optional specifier that may be coded only after having diagnosed and coded severity and trait domains. Another significant change was that the diagnostic features for the Borderline pattern were no longer those known from ICD-10 – emotionally unstable Personality Disorder, borderline type – but instead a slight revision of the criteria in the American Psychiatric Association's (2013) *Diagnostic and Statistical Manual of Mental Disorders* (5th ed.; *DSM-5*) classification. In addition to the inclusion of the borderline pattern, the working group also decided that the ICD-11 model should include a more exhaustive description of self-functioning on par with interpersonal functioning, which had previously been the primary focus (Huprich, 2020; Huprich et al., 2018; Reed, 2018).

It may be important to be aware of the fact that if you read empirical literature about ICD-11 Personality Disorders published before 2017, findings may be based on previous proposals for the classification and thus be outdated compared to the now official version.

At the time of writing, there seems to be growing international acceptance and interest in the new ICD-11 approach (Chanen et al., 2022; Prevolnik Rupel et al., 2021; Sharp & Oldham, 2023; Widiger et al., 2024). It is expected that European countries will be first movers in implementing the system (Bach et al., 2022).

Leaving the Traditional Categories

Where previously we have classified Personality Disorder based on categories of distinct types (e.g., avoidant, borderline, dependent), we now have to get used to classifying based on levels of severity (mild, moderate, severe). This continuum from mild to severe is also referred to as a *dimensional* approach because it is a dimension of severity. In contrast to ICD-10's and DSM-5's focus on "counting criteria" for each type of Personality Disorder (i.e., polythetic approach), the ICD-11 will focus on general diagnostic requirements and features of Personality Disorder (see Table 1.1).

This change should be seen in light of the fact that WHO, based on 30 years of research, has sought to do away with criteria-based diagnostics, where diagnoses are defined somewhat rigidly based on a given number of criteria met with a fixed, but pseudo-accurate threshold. For example, ICD-10's diagnostic criteria for F60.5 Anankastic Personality Disorder means that two people can fulfil the criteria for the diagnosis without having a single symptom in common. In everyday life, two people may actually experience the disorder very differently based on the individual composition of criteria met (e.g., doubt and caution in one and rigidity and stubbornness in the other). This is one of the reasons why ICD-11's diagnostic descriptions are not as definitive or fixed in language but can be flexibly applied to better match the diverse clinical reality that exists.

Understanding a diagnosis as distinct from other diagnoses is particularly meaningful for medical conditions. A broken leg is different from appendicitis, heart disease is different from kidney disease, and the treatments for such different conditions will often be very different (e.g., surgery or medication).

Diagnoses for mental disorders do not describe such well-defined diseases or syndromes with a clear separation between cause (e.g., viral infection) and symptoms (e.g., cough). Knowledge about the exact causes of mental disorders, including Personality Disorders, is still very limited, which is why it is not so easy to separate cause and symptom. The multifactorial origin of mental disorders means that any particular risk factor (e.g., a specific adverse event) may lead to different or no disorder (multifinality), and that different risk factors may lead to the same disorder (equifinality). In other words, we cannot reliably link the diagnosis to specific causes (e.g., trauma) or solutions (e.g., therapy). This issue is well recognised in the classification of mental disorders in general but is arguably particularly pronounced when it comes to Personality Disorder (Kendler et al., 2011).

Until the introduction of ICD-11, the diagnosis of Personality Disorder has been based on a categorical understanding with a total of eight specific types, in addition to the possibility of diagnosing "Other specific personality disorder" (e.g., narcissistic or passive-aggressive) or an unspecified or mixed type. As mentioned, over the past 30–40 years, research has documented significant problems with a categorical classification of Personality Disorders (Frances, 1980; Skodol, 2014; Widiger & Trull, 2007), which we briefly summarise in the following four sections.

Extensive Diagnostic Overlap

When patients are systematically screened for ICD-10 Personality Disorder, the most common picture is that they fulfil criteria for at least two or more Personality Disorders simultaneously. In particular, the borderline diagnosis co-occurs with virtually all other types of Personality Disorder (Karterud et al., 2003). This suggests that there are a number of characteristics or problems that cut across the different diagnoses. The ICD-11 does not allow for co-occurrence among different Personality Disorder diagnoses as it is simply not possible to have two different levels of severity at the same time (e.g., having a Mild and a Severe Personality Disorder at the same time). Thus, the starting point is that people with Personality Disorder struggle with a number of the same general problems (e.g., self-esteem, relationship issues, and emotion regulation), and that the diverse and overlapping presence of these problems is not a matter of what has traditionally been called co-occurrence or "co-morbidity," but rather is an expression of different degrees and manifestations of one and the same fundamental disorder.

Heterogeneity Within Diagnostic Categories

With a number of defined criteria and a set threshold for how many criteria must be met, Personality Disorders in ICD-10 and DSM-5 can be combined in hundreds of ways. As a result, individuals with the same diagnosis can be very different, which can cause problems both in pointing to a clear-cut treatment model and in identifying specific causal relationships. In practice, two people may fulfil the diagnostic criteria for an Anankastic Personality Disorder without having a single symptom in common. With ICD-11, it is possible to describe this heterogeneity more systematically, both in terms of overall severity and specific trait expressions. For example, there will be a significant difference between a person who is characterised by Negative Affectivity alone and a person who has prominent traits of both Negative Affectivity and Disinhibition (see Chapters 5 and 6).

Pseudo-Accurate Diagnostic Thresholds

The ICD-10 and DSM-5 diagnostic approach specifies a number of criteria that must be met in order to make a diagnosis (e.g., four out of seven criteria for Avoidant Personality Disorder). However, a key problem here is that these thresholds have generally not been empirically determined or the scientific foundation is questionable. This means that there is no significant difference between people who fulfil four or five criteria for Borderline Personality Disorder. In addition to the problems with the arbitrary threshold, it is also clear that the categorical understanding, where a given phenomenon is either present or not, involves a significant loss of information. For example, extensive sub-diagnostic data are lost when reducing the information to either "disordered" or "healthy." With ICD-11, the clinician decides whether personality functioning is disturbed to a mild, moderate, or severe degree and the clinician is also allowed to specify sub-diagnostic Personality Difficulty. This is not determined on the basis of a fixed number of criteria, but instead depends on a global assessment, which can be thought of as a "matching process" in which the clinician compares phenomenological descriptions with the diagnostic features and examples for Mild, Moderate, and Severe Personality Disorder, respectively. This diagnostic process thus has more in common with a holistic identification of a "gestalt" or "prototype." Anything else in this context would be considered pseudo-accurate, meaning something that sounds precise on the surface but, in reality, covers a wide spectrum of diversity. Interestingly, research indicates that a severity continuum rather than a categorical Personality Disorder diagnosis creates less public stigma (Stricker et al., 2024).

Unspecified Diagnosis and General Underdiagnosis of Personality Disorder

Several studies have shown that unspecified Personality Disorder is the most commonly made diagnosis besides Borderline and Dissocial Personality Disorder (Pedersen & Simonsen, 2014; Tyrer et al., 2019). This diagnosis is inherently inadequate on its own, as it simply specifies that something is wrong, but does not indicate the degree or nature of the problem. It can carry a significant risk of stigmatisation and has little guiding potential for both the clinician and the diagnosed person. With ICD-11, it is still possible to diagnose Personality Disorder without specifying the severity. In this case, however, it must still be confirmed that the general diagnostic requirements are met (see "General Diagnostic Requirements" in Chapter 2). In many countries the problems with the categorical diagnosis of Personality Disorder, including the inability to tier and specify the diagnosis, have led to Personality Difficulty and Disorders generally being underdiagnosed and actually occurring with decreasing frequency. For example, in Danish mental health services the diagnosis is made for approximately 10–12% of patients (Pedersen & Simonsen, 2014), while international research suggests that it is present in more than half of psychiatric patients (Alnæs & Torgersen, 1988; Beckwith et al., 2014). This can be seen as particularly problematic in relation to an ideal of adequate and tailored treatment.

Focus on Clinical Utility

An important overall aim of ICD-11 has been to increase the clinical utility of the classification (Reed, 2010), which is particularly relevant for the rather complex area of Personality Disorders (Bach & First, 2018; Pan & Wang, 2024). Clinical utility can be described as the "third pillar" of diagnostic classification, alongside reliability and validity. There is not complete agreement on all components of the definition of clinical utility, but most definitions emphasise the practical aspects, that is, the extent to which a diagnosis is easy to use and, not least, easy to communicate to others, whether it is the person being diagnosed or colleagues, relatives, or carers. In addition, clinical utility often emphasises the extent to which the diagnosis is useful in clinical decision-making processes and provides useful information about the prognosis of the disorder. Studies have shown that clinicians are generally in favour of a dimensional approach to diagnoses (Bernstein et al. 2007; Brown et al., 2023; Evans et al., 2013; Morey & Hopwood, 2019; Reed et al., 2011). For example, Reed and colleagues (2011) found that two out of three psychiatrists prefer a system that is flexible and guiding rather than based on strict criteria for diagnoses. In addition, they found that up to 90% of psychiatrists favour a significantly fewer number of diagnoses (with around 100 diagnoses rated as the most useful), and that around 70% of psychiatrists believe that diagnoses should incorporate dimensional components. A similar pattern was found among psychologists from around the world (Evans et al., 2013).

A Danish study has shown that professionals generally find the ICD-11 classification of Personality Disorders more clinically useful than ICD-10, at least in terms of treatment planning, communication with patients, and ease of use (Hansen et al., 2019). However, for communicating with other professionals or describing the patient's personality as a whole, there were no significant differences in usability. A similar pattern was found in a study among psychiatrists and psychologists in New Zealand (Brown et al., 2023).

Describing and understanding psychopathology on a continuum of severity provides the best opportunities for more precise and individualised treatment, such as adjusting the treatment dose according to the severity of the disorder (Hopwood et al., 2020). In addition, research also shows that a dimensional understanding of mental disorders may reduce the tendency for stigmatising attitudes among people working with assessment and treatment of people with Personality Disorders (Peter et al., 2021; Stricker et al., 2024).

Chapter 2
General Diagnostic Practice

In this chapter, we attempt to cover all the essentials for clinicians in connection with using the new classification. The chapter begins with a crash course in how the basic concepts of "personality functioning" and "trait domains" can be applied in practice. We then focus on the general diagnostic requirements, distinguishing between "disorder" and sub-diagnostic "difficulty." Finally, a number of important differential diagnostic considerations and developmental aspects are discussed, as well as how to deal with co-occurring mental disorders.

Crash Course in the Clinical Use of Personality Functioning and Trait Domains

Understanding a patient's personality can be the key to a deeper and more comprehensive conceptualization and treatment of their mental health problems. Using the ICD-11 classification of Personality Disorder and Related Traits, we take as our starting point a set of core human capacities that underpin mental health. Regardless of the diagnostic framework or therapeutic approach, treatment can be organised using these psychological capacities and manifestations, which together are called personality functioning (see Table 2.1).

For example, most clinicians will recognise how patients' problematic ways of seeing themselves and others will manifest in the therapeutic relationship. Sometimes we may be unsure of how best to interact with the patient in a meaningful way, and their needs may seem overwhelming or confusing to us. We may feel pressured to overstep our own professional boundaries and become too invested in the patient's problems and behaviours. Depending on our theoretical frame of understanding, we may refer to such common phenomena as transference and countertransference, therapeutic resistance, "chemistry," therapy-interfering behaviour, therapeutic rapport, and alliance rupture. For example, we may experience moments where we are unable to think clearly

Table 2.1   Abbreviated overview of aspects that contribute to the assessment of personality functioning

Personality functioning	
Aspects of the self	**Interpersonal functioning**
• Sense of identity (too loose or fixed) • Self-esteem (inflated or deflated) • Self-perception (strengths and weaknesses) • Self-direction (too weak or rigid)	• Engagement in relationships (avoidance or desperation) • Perspective-taking (too little or too much) • Mutuality in relationships (give and take) • Conflict management (submissive or aggressive)
Manifestations		
Emotional	**Cognitive**	**Behaviour**
• Experience and expression • Over- or underreactive • Recognising own emotions	• Reality testing • Decision making • Stability and flexibility of beliefs	• Too little/much self-control • Harm to self • Harm to others
Global psychosocial impairment and/or distress		
Personal, family, social, educational, employment, or other significant functioning		

and our emotional reactions cloud our judgement and decisions. We can get caught in counterproductive interactions that we do not know how to get out of, or, worse, do not even realise we are in. We can get caught up in power struggles characterised by themes of dominance and submissiveness. At times, the clinician perceives a distance towards the patient or an urge to say "pull yourself together" or to overprotect and carry the patient through life. These types of experiences in the clinician can often reflect important aspects about the patient's self and interpersonal functioning and recognising them may be crucial in helping clinicians build a functioning alliance and adjust their therapeutic approach, which is usually a prerequisite for effective treatment.

A concrete example of a clinical issue might be a patient whose impaired or dysregulated self-esteem is the driving force behind an unhealthy dependency on recognition from others or an inner self-criticism that leads to perfectionism, stress, anxiousness, and sadness. Compromised self-esteem can also underlie an overt sense of shame or overcompensatory self-aggrandisement. People with this kind of personality dysfunction may tend to avoid others because being around them triggers feelings of inadequacy, or they may use another type of avoidance behaviour, such as drugs or aggression, to keep their own feelings or other people at a distance. Most people who work in clinical practice encounter people with these kinds of personality issues.

As a consequence of difficulties related to aspects of the self, patients may have problems with the way they perceive and relate to other people. For example, their idea of what others think may be driven by their own sense of inferiority or self-insecurities. To put it simply, what really belongs to the person is wrongly attributed to someone else. In practice, this can manifest itself as a tendency to feel critically observed by other people and a belief that others think negatively about you. In general, such patterns can cause a lot of confusion in communicating with other people, including relationships with healthcare professionals. The patient may be trapped in a dogmatic, distrustful, or hostile perception, which can include being vigilant for any sign that we do not like them, wish to hurt them, or abandon them (e.g., when we are late or have to cancel an appointment). If we as practitioners do not have a language for such issues, we can end up enacting or becoming exactly what the patient fears in the treatment process.

Due to the above-mentioned dysfunctions in aspects of the self and relationships with other people, the patient will typically also have problems with their emotional life. Specifically, this can be problems with containing and regulating the difficult emotions that arise when a negative view of oneself and other people is a controlling factor. Some patients tend to disconnect themselves from difficult emotions so they cannot feel or "listen" to them. Others may be prone to becoming overwhelmed by the emotions and react with aggression, impulsive self-destructive behaviour, or self-harm. There may also be a lack of ability to recognise difficult emotions or acknowledge unwanted emotions (e.g., sadness or anger), which is probably familiar to many professionals under the term Alexithymia. The latter can result in the patient being unaware of the thoughts and feelings behind their own destructive actions, and they struggle to express their emotional states in a healthy way. Such aspects of disordered personality functioning tend to perpetuate the patient's problems and complicate treatment.

Alignment with Psychotherapy Models

The naturally intertwined aspects of self and interpersonal functioning will be obvious to many clinicians. Psychodynamic clinicians may think of internal models of self and others (e.g., object relations), whereas proponents of cognitive behavioural therapy may link it to the patient's core beliefs about self and others. For example, a patient may hold negative beliefs about the self ("I am inferior and stupid"), which play out interpersonally ("I must avoid other people so they don't realise how useless I am"). Thus, using cognitive behavioural therapy to modify the patient's negative core beliefs can also be expected to promote both a healthier self and better interpersonal functioning. Similarly, mentalisation-based therapy works to strengthen the patient's ability to understand mental states in themselves and others. Schema therapy can focus on early developed schemas in relation to oneself (e.g., "I am defective") and other people (e.g., "others will let me down or mistreat me") as well as various self-states ("modes") of activated schemas and coping responses. In emotion-focused therapy, the focus is on emotions as the key to self-understanding along with patterns of interpersonal interaction. In intensive short-term dynamic psychotherapy, anxieties about inner conflicts and emotions (aspects of the self) and about relationships and intimacy (interpersonal functioning) are typically addressed. Finally, proponents of dialectical behavioural therapy can facilitate similar processes by working on the patient's self-regulation and relationship skills.

Severity of Problems

Overall, the assessment of personality functioning covers both well-functioning and dysfunctional personality, allowing us to determine the patient's level of personality functioning on a continuum ranging from healthy functioning to Severe Personality Disorder (see Table 2.2). These severity levels are often good indications of the intensity and extent of treatment that needs to be initiated, which we will describe in more detail in Chapter 6.

Personality Traits

While personality functioning points to the overall severity of a patient's difficulties, the patient's specific composition of personality traits can be said to portray the individual's dispositional expression of these disturbances. Personality traits describe essential aspects of the patient's basic temperament. For example, normal Introversion and Extroversion are reflected as high or low levels of Detachment, while a natural sensitivity is expressed under Negative Affectivity. However, because it is all about personality pathology, ICD-11 emphasises only the maladaptive expression of the personality style. There

Table 2.2 Levels of personality functioning for specific impairments in self-esteem and understanding others

Level	
0. Healthy functioning	Have a stable and positive self-esteem with an overall accurate understanding of the experience of others.
1. Personality difficulty	Self-esteem is sometimes characterised by a distorted view of oneself, while the ability to realistically understand the experience of others can be slightly problematic.
2. Mild disorder	Self-esteem is vulnerable (e.g., they have difficulty recovering from experiences where self-esteem has been injured), while the ability to understand the experience of others is problematic.
3. Moderate disorder	Significant problems maintaining a stable positive self-esteem (e.g., has an unrealistically negative or positive view of themselves), while the ability to understand the experience of others is significantly impaired.
4. Severe disorder	Severe problems with self-esteem regulation (e.g., self-loathing or grandiosity), while there is a markedly compromised ability to consider and understand the experience or motivation of others.

is also no doubt that these maladaptive expressions of personality traits also reflect dysfunctional patterns of coping, such as pronounced Detachment (e.g., avoidance of perceived criticism from others) and perfectionism (e.g., overcompensation for sense of inferiority). Thus, it makes a significant difference whether a patient with Moderate Personality Disorder is characterised by Negative Affectivity and Detachment (e.g., overly anxious, inhibited, and avoidant) or Dissociality and Disinhibition (e.g., self-centred, dominant, and reckless). These two different combinations of trait domains reflect different kinds of problems and point to different interventions. The importance of specifying the trait domains in question becomes even more apparent when dealing with the specific problems that apply to each trait domain. As described in Appendix B of this book, the different facets of the trait domains can be systematically portrayed using the Five-Factor Inventory for ICD-11 (FFiCD; Oltmanns & Widiger, 2020) or a specific scoring key of the Personality Inventory for DSM-5 (Bach et al., 2017; Sellbom et al., 2020). In addition to the five trait domains, FFiCD also describes 20 underlying facets and 47 nuances. For example, facets from Negative Affectivity (e.g., shame), Anankastia (e.g., perfectionism), and Dissociality (e.g., self-centredness), as well as nuances such as separation anxiety, rigidity, and entitlement, respectively, can help guide clinicians on how to best establish an alliance with the patient and what they can expect to work with as a therapist.

Clinical Use of Both Personality Functioning and Trait Domains

Although personality traits describe individual expressions, they are not sufficient to provide a clinically useful portrait of a patient's Personality Disorder. Personality traits describe essential aspects of *who* we are and *how* we behave, but do not explain *why* we act the way we do. For example, the infamous American serial killer Ted Bundy was thought to be characterised by personality traits such as Dissociality, Anankastia, and Negative Affectivity (Samuel & Widiger, 2007). Indeed, a similar pattern characterises many successful politicians (Scott & Medeiros, 2020). Therefore, to understand key aspects of personality and Personality Disorder, we also need to understand aspects of personality functioning, such as the ability to perceive and appreciate the perspective of others, the ability to develop and maintain close and mutually satisfying relationships, and the ability to select, plan, and realise appropriate goals. For the same reason, personality functioning has been referred to as the language of psychotherapy (Hutsebaut, 2023). Therefore, personality functioning forms the basis for the assessment, diagnosis, and classification of Personality Disorder, while trait domains are merely a specification of it, which is optional.

Personality is fundamentally about questions like "Who am I?" and "How do I want to share my life with others?" (Sharp & Wall, 2021). These questions are dynamic and only make sense from a developmental perspective. Personality Disorder occurs when the "answers" to the aforementioned questions continue to be problematic in life. The essence of this problem lies in personality functioning itself and not in the trait description. Personality traits show up very early in children, but we do not describe them as having a Personality Disorder because the traits do not adequately tell us anything about who the person is and how they want to share their life with others.

When we as clinicians prepare a treatment and do case formulation, we can use the patient's personality functioning as a starting point to understand their vulnerability "from the inside," while personality traits can provide a more stylistic description of these vulnerabilities and disorders "from the outside." In other words, personality functioning can be said to capture how our patients generally manage themselves and their relationships, while the trait domains further portray the dysfunction that got the patients referred to your clinic.

In addition to treatment planning and case formulation, assessment and classification of personality functioning can also be used dynamically to track clinical progress ("tracking"), while trait domains are more likely to remain stable over time. This is because personality traits tend to be more resistant to change, which is because they reflect our biological temperament to some extent, whereas personality functioning is more malleable (Hopwood, Donnellan et al., 2011; Hopwood, Malone et al., 2011; Kiel, Hopwood et al., 2024; Roche, 2018; Wright et al., 2016). For example, after a longer course of treatment, a patient may change diagnosis from Moderate to Mild Personality Disorder, while the presence of Negative Affectivity and Detachment still characterises the patient. As clinicians, we should therefore focus our attention on *understanding* the patient's personality traits while seeking to *change* the overall personality functioning. However, the picture is not quite as straightforward as certain aspects of trait domains may also reflect embedded coping patterns such as Detachment (e.g., emotional withdrawal) and Anankastia (e.g., perfectionism), making the maladaptive trait domains more malleable than what is commonly found in similar traits such as Introversion (e.g., quiet and introspective) and Conscientiousness (e.g., meticulous and orderly). In this way, ICD-11 trait domains can be modified to some extent by therapeutic work with the patient's dysfunctional coping strategies.

Overall, assessment and classification of severity can be used to determine the intensity and extent of the intervention required, whereas trait domains can be used to determine the focus and style of treatment. For example, trait domains can provide a better understanding of individual triggers and stressors that can provoke and amplify the patient's problems (e.g., Negative Affectivity in the form of distrust and emotional lability), thereby also indicating how practitioners can interact with and establish the best possible relationship with the patient. For more in-depth guidance on clinical work, please refer to Chapter 6.

General Diagnostic Requirements

The first and most crucial thing we as clinicians need to consider is whether the general diagnostic requirements for a Personality Disorder apply. It is worth noting that the overall determination of whether a Personality

Disorder is diagnosed remains a categorical decision, where the overall categorisation in itself does not indicate the severity of the disorder. In the following bullet points, the necessary essential characteristics (requirements) of a Personality Disorder are described:

- An enduring disturbance characterised by problems in functioning of aspects of the self (e.g., identity, self-worth, accuracy of self-view, self-direction), and/or interpersonal dysfunction (e.g., ability to develop and maintain close and mutually satisfying relationships, ability to understand others' perspectives and to manage conflict in relationships).
- The disturbance has persisted over an extended period of time (e.g., lasting 2 years or more).
- The disturbance is manifest in patterns of cognition, emotional experience, emotional expression, and behaviour that are maladaptive (e.g., inflexible or poorly regulated).
- The disturbance is manifest across a range of personal and social situations (i.e., is not limited to specific relationships or social roles), though it may be consistently evoked by particular types of circumstances and not others.
- The symptoms are not due to the direct effects of a medication or substance, including withdrawal effects, and are not better accounted for by another mental disorder, a disease of the nervous system, or another medical condition.
- The disturbance is associated with substantial distress or significant impairment in personal, family, social, educational, occupational, or other important areas of functioning.
- Personality Disorder should not be diagnosed if the patterns of behaviour characterising the personality disturbance are developmentally appropriate (e.g., problems related to establishing an independent self-identity during adolescence) or can be explained primarily by social or cultural factors, including socio-political conflict.

(World Health Organization, 2024, pp. 554–555)

For a clinician, a good indication of a possible Personality Disorder will often be that the patient has had difficulties over a long period of time and to an extent that it has caused problems across different situations. Perhaps the person has felt inferior for as long as they can remember or has always had many conflicts with others.

A new feature of the ICD-11 classification is that the personality disturbances must not necessarily have been stably present since childhood or early adolescence, as long as they have generally been present over a longer period of time. This makes it possible to diagnose patients at a later age ("late onset" Personality Disorder), even if no significant dysfunction can be identified in childhood and adolescence. On the other hand, there will usually have been some degree of maladaptive patterns or vulnerabilities earlier in life (i.e., prodromal Personality Disorder).

When assessing dysfunctional patterns in cognition, emotional life, and behaviour, it is essential to consider the areas specified in Table 3.1 (Chapter 3), which form the basis for making a diagnosis and determining the severity of the diagnosis. At the same time, however, it is important to emphasise that one should not be blinded by the written diagnostic definitions but, instead, remember that these descriptions are there to help the clinician in the assessment, where the personality must always be seen in context. Generally, the clinical descriptions and diagnostic requirements should not be used as a fixed manual for clinical assessment. Instead, the clinician is urged to use their broader understanding of psychopathology and clinical competencies learned through appropriate education, training, and experience. The experienced clinician recognises that a valid assessment is less about the specific content, such as the person having experienced feelings of inferiority, but more about the fact that a given problem is pervasive and not exclusively affected by specific circumstances. We will often talk about a rigidity in the disturbed personality, which can be contrasted with the flexibility that is often present in people with a healthy functioning personality. If the personality problems only appear in very limited contexts and are of short duration, ICD-11 clearly points out that the clinician must then consider whether it is instead a more or less normal response to the given circumstances. In such cases, it is usually more relevant for the clinician to look towards the specific difficulties that occur in relationships and situations than to make a diagnosis.

The general requirements also include some exclusion requirements to ensure that a misdiagnosis is not made in cases where a given symptom pattern can be fully explained by other conditions or solely attributed to other diagnoses. This requirement is further elaborated under a heading in the classification describing boundaries with other disorders and conditions (differential diagnosis). It should be noted that throughout the ICD-11 classification, co-occurring diagnoses are generally allowed without stronger recommendations against diagnosing two particular disorders together. Instead, it is recognised that a number of persistent disorders (e.g., Autism Spectrum Disorder [ASD], Schizotypal Disorder, Complex Post Traumatic Stress Disorder, and Dissociative Identity Disorder) share features similar to Personality Disorder. It is specifically pointed out that an additional diagnosis of Personality Disorder should typically not be assigned unless additional personality features are present that contribute to significant problems and cannot fully be accounted for by the presence of the mental disorder in question (e.g., ASD). This is often a matter of careful clinical judgement and will be further elaborated on the following pages. Finally, there must be significant distress and/or psychosocial impairment before a diagnosis can be made at all. Once a clinician believes that a person appears to fulfil the general requirements, the next step in the process is to determine severity, using Table 3.1 (Chapter 3) as a starting point, combined with specific definitions and examples of the different severity levels (Chapter 4).

Is It a Disorder or Just a Difficulty?

When it comes down to it, clinicians can consider the description of Mild Personality Disorder as a guideline for when a Personality Disorder may be present, as the personality disturbances must be at least mild in order for the diagnosis to be applied. Sometimes it can be a difficult task to determine whether it is a Personality Disorder at all or merely a sub-diagnostic Personality Difficulty, which is quite common in the population and not least in our patients. In fact, research suggests that only a minority of about 12–23% of the general population have no personality problems at all (Bach et al., 2023; Yang et al., 2010). For a more detailed description of the ICD-11 definition of sub-diagnostic Personality Disorder, see Chapter 4.

An easy rule of thumb is the three Ps, which stand for *pathological*, *persistent*, and *pervasive*. These three characteristic aspects can thus guide clinicians in considering whether personality difficulties are more normal than abnormal, more adaptive than maladaptive, more periodic ("state") than habitual ("trait"), and more contextual than pervasive. At the same time, clinicians must never forget that subthreshold Personality Difficulty can have significant clinical and prognostic significance (Karukivi et al., 2017; Morgan et al., 2013; Zimmerman et al., 2013).

Differential Diagnosis

Personality Disorder has at times been a differential diagnostic minefield, where one can very easily misstep and, in fairness, be confronted with advocates of other major diagnostic groups, such as the schizophrenia spectrum (Zandersen & Parnas, 2019), the autism spectrum (Rinaldi et al., 2021), Attention Deficit Hyperactivity Disorder (ADHD; Tiger et al., 2022), Bipolar Type II Disorder (Smith et al., 2004), and, not least, complex PTSD (Felding et al., 2021). There has also traditionally been no consensus on whether a Personality Disorder should be diagnosed at the same time as another "heavy" disorder such as Schizophrenia (Simonsen & Newton-Howes, 2018). We will now highlight key differential diagnostic considerations based on the guidelines that now officially appear in ICD-11.

As a starting point, a variety of mental disorders can be characterised by enduring disturbances in cognition, emotional experience, and behaviour that manifest across personal and social situations and are associated with significant impairment in aspects of the self (e.g., self-esteem and goal-directedness) and/or interpersonal dysfunction (e.g., ability to develop and maintain close and mutually satisfying relationships, to understand others' perspectives, and to manage conflict in relationships). Individuals with these disorders can thus also be considered to fulfil the diagnostic criteria for a Personality Disorder. But let us pause here for a moment and carefully consider the ICD-11 guidelines. In general, individuals with such disorders should not be further diagnosed with a Personality Disorder unless there are significant personality disturbances that cannot be attributed to the disorder in question or that exceed what one would expect to see in the disorder in question. As previously described, ICD-11 has done away with strict criteria-based diagnostics based on pseudo-accurate thresholds. This means that it pragmatically allows more room for professional judgement in a clinical reality characterised by complexity and nuance. ICD-11 thus clarifies that even when the aforementioned premises do not apply, there may be specific situations where an additional diagnosis of Personality Disorder may be warranted. For example, this may apply to situations where it is assessed that a patient will benefit from a specific treatment that requires a diagnosis of Personality Disorder. In other words, the World Health Organization's vision of alleviating suffering is a factor that can, in practice, override and "overrule" general diagnostic guidelines, providing greater differential diagnostic leeway. But here, of course, it becomes crucial to have a solid knowledge of the symptoms and characteristics of other persistent mental disorders before it can be decided whether additional problems may actually be attributed to Personality Disorder and whether treatment for personality dysfunction could be beneficial. The latter can occur, for example, in people diagnosed with recurrent or persistent depression, where several forms of treatment have been tried without sufficient effect. In this case, it is our belief that a Personality Disorder diagnosis could be assigned for a person with sub-diagnostic difficulty, if this diagnosis could in fact help the person get a relevant evidence-based treatment (e.g., psychotherapy).

We will now highlight key considerations of differential diagnoses in terms of ASD, Schizotypal Disorder, Bipolar Disorder, complex PTSD, secondary

Personality Disorder, ADHD, Dissociative Identity Disorder, Dysthymic Disorder, Separation Anxiety Disorder, Social Anxiety Disorder, Obsessive-Compulsive Disorder (OCD), Conduct-Dissocial Disorder, substance abuse and dependence, and impulse control disorders in general.

Autism Spectrum Disorder (ASD)

Individuals with ASD may have difficulties in establishing and maintaining relationships as well as challenges with identity and emotion regulation in a way that is similar to the difficulties seen in Personality Disorder. In people with ASD, such issues are usually due to sensory hypersensitivity, often combined with a deficient sense of social communication and social interaction (e.g., decoding social interaction). In people with Personality Disorder, on the other hand, there may be more of a reduced frustration tolerance, poor conflict management, and fear of rejection or abandonment. These differences and similarities will be elaborated on with the purpose of providing clinical guidance for differential diagnosis (Bach & Vestergaard, 2023).

Many people with autism and normal intellectual functioning may have had a seemingly unremarkable childhood and schooling due to their adaptability, overcompensation, and "masking" of difficulties. However, due to sensory hypersensitivity to sound, light, smell, texture, temperature, and mood, combined with inevitable experiences of failure (e.g., bullying due to misunderstandings in communication with classmates and unclear environmental demands), psychological stressors may accumulate over time, leading to a pattern of meltdowns and mental disorders. Personality Disorder and ASD are similar in that both disorders typically manifest during puberty and both diagnoses have a high co-occurrence of anxiety, depression, self-harm, and eating disorders. In ASD, symptoms are more related to sensory and change sensitivity and self-harm is more likely to be driven by accumulated stress that has led to a "meltdown" (Jadav & Bal, 2022).

People with Personality Disorder typically have a history of neglect or abuse growing up, so they may have a heightened sensitivity or sensitivity to signs of rejection, abandonment, or insults. Such unfavourable childhood experiences can also characterise people with undiagnosed ASD, as they have repeatedly experienced being misunderstood, exploited, and traumatised by meltdowns, while also feeling socially excluded and alienated.

In both ASD and Personality Disorder, there are examples of hypomentalisation (i.e., reading too little into social interactions and not understanding others' perspectives) as well as hyper-mentalisation (i.e., reading too much into social situations and thinking too much about others' perspectives). Remarkably, hyper-mentalisation can be highly prevalent in girls or women with ASD who throughout life have compensated for and masked their difficulties by paying extra attention to decoding interactions and social information (Isaksson et al., 2019; Vegni et al., 2021), which can ultimately result in burnout, meltdown, breakdown, shutdown, self-harm, and suicidal behaviour, which can resemble the emotional dysregulation, dissociation, and self-harm we often see in Personality Disorder (Arnold et al., 2023; Darling Rasmussen, 2023). Clinicians should therefore be particularly aware that individuals with ASD can often function unobtrusively in many contexts, using masking and camouflaging to such an extent that the disorder goes "under the radar" and is overlooked by professionals (Bradley et al., 2021). Nevertheless, it should also be recognised that camouflaging or masking is currently not very well understood and may at times also be seen as an adaptive and necessary strategy (Cook et al., 2021; Fombonne, 2020).

People with ASD can exhibit a form of social naivety and literal understanding of other people's statements that may result in them being taken advantage of or subjugated, which can be confused with some of the interpersonal issues seen in Personality Disorder. The repeated experiences of being used, deceived, and ridiculed by others can also lead to a pattern of trust issues and withdrawal, which can also be seen in Personality Disorder.

As previously mentioned, girls and women with ASD in particular can appear inconspicuous in contact because they use masking, which can ultimately have a detrimental effect on their mental health and lead to repeated severe stress reactions and meltdowns including transient psychotic features, which can also be seen in Severe Personality Disorder under affective arousal. Finally, rigid thinking is often present in people with ASD, which can be confused with the black-and-white thinking that often occurs in Personality Disorder.

Girls and women with ASD may be so focused on fitting in with their surroundings ("chameleon behaviour") that they may struggle to find their own role and identity in life, which in turn can be confused with the more pervasive identity issues that often characterise Personality Disorder. Unlike the challenges with social roles and identity associated with ASD, identity issues in Personality Disorder are more pervasive, with distinctly shifting interests, values, and goals. For example, a person with Personality Disorder may adopt the interests of others in order to gain their recognition, while people with ASD will typically hold uncompromisingly to their own interests and values. However, the latter can make it challenging to distinguish ASD from a Personality Disorder with predominant Anankastia, where the goal-directedness can also be inflexible. Finally, ASD is mainly perceived as innate and therefore usually manifests in childhood or at the latest in early adolescence, while Personality Disorder is not innate and usually first appears in adolescence.

In summary, it can be difficult to distinguish ASD and Personality Disorder from each other because both diagnoses have a pervasive and persistent nature that relates to aspects of self and interpersonal functioning. However, people with ASD may be distinguished by having sensory disturbances (i.e., sensing too much or too little), using self-stimulatory behaviour ("stimming"), being uncompromisingly honest even when it is not beneficial, having special interests, being prone to misunderstand sarcasm and irony, finding eye contact unnatural or strenuous, having a high need for alone time after socialising ("downtime"), and often using imitation or neutral facial expressions. Crucially, people with ASD often have persistent, restricted, repetitive, and inflexible patterns of behaviour, interests, or activities that have been present since childhood. It should be noted, however, that special interests and patterns may be less pronounced or appear normal and socially acceptable, especially in girls (e.g., horses, fantasy literature, film, fashion design, psychology, social relationships), which is why it is important to identify how these interests function as well as their quality and intensity. If the diagnostic requirements for ASD are met, this diagnosis will usually override and overrule a Personality Disorder. However, as with the other ICD-11 diagnoses, there may be clinical circumstances where it makes sense to supplement the diagnosis with a Personality Disorder. Just as people outside the autism spectrum can develop a Personality Disorder, people within the autism spectrum can of course also develop a Personality Disorder.

Schizotypal Disorder

Like Personality Disorder, Schizotypal Disorder is also characterised by a lasting disturbance in the person's way of interpreting and experiencing themselves, other people, and the world, resulting in maladaptive patterns of emotional expression and behaviour resulting in significant problems in functioning (e.g., self-referential, anxious, and distrustful ideas with a tendency to social withdrawal).

However, individuals with Schizotypal Disorder should not be diagnosed with a concurrent Personality Disorder based on problems that are solely a consequence of the symptoms of Schizotypal Disorder. If additional problematic aspects of personality dysfunction are present (e.g., tendency to harm others or to submit to others in a harmful way) and contribute to significant problems in interpersonal functioning, it may sometimes be appropriate to also diagnose Personality Disorder. This is the case, for example, if it is felt that the person may benefit from a treatment programme tailored to people with a Personality Disorder. However, it must be acknowledged that clinical reality will always be full of grey areas, and that ICD-11 thus also exemplifies that people with a Severe Personality Disorder may in some cases have a highly eccentric self-view without meeting the diagnostic requirements for a Schizotypal Disorder.

Bipolar Disorder and Cyclothymia

Like Personality Disorder, Bipolar Type II Disorder can also include impulsive behaviour (e.g., impulse buying or impulsive sexual activity) and unstable or fluctuating states of affect. However, Personality Disorder does not by itself involve depressive, hypomanic, manic, or mixed episodes. In addition, affect lability and impulsivity in Personality Disorder are often reactions to circumstances (e.g., a desperate affect response with impulsive behaviour to the experience of being belittled or the fear of being abandoned). Furthermore, manic symptoms of increased self-confidence can easily be confused with excessive positive self-esteem and overestimation of own strengths as can be seen in Personality Disorder. Similarly, reckless risk-taking behaviour in mania can easily be mistaken for a Personality Disorder with predominant Dissociality and Disinhibition. In manic and hypomanic episodes, there is less of a reactive or interpersonal component and symptoms are triggered independently of the immediate circumstances around the person. However, general stressors (e.g., lack of sleep and adversity) are often contributing factors to a manic episode. Finally, ICD-11 also allows for a specification of "rapid cycling," where mood can alternate between depression and hypomania over the course of a day, which can sometimes be confused with affect lability in Personality Disorder. The same can be said for cyclothymia, where the affective instability has a lower intensity than in Bipolar Disorder. When it comes down to it, it is not surprising that the differential diagnosis here is challenging, as cyclothymia has traditionally been categorised as a Cyclothymic Personality Disorder, cf., ICD-7 to ICD-9 (Pull, 2014).

However, it should also be emphasised that Personality Disorder and Bipolar Disorder co-occur relatively frequently (25–40%) (Sletved et al., 2023). Therefore, both diagnoses can be made simultaneously if the diagnostic requirements are met. This would also apply to cyclothymia. However, it is recommended to investigate symptoms of Personality Disorder as far as possible while the patient is neither in a manic nor in an acute phase of a Depressive Episode.

Complex PTSD

Like Personality Disorder, complex PTSD can also be characterised by a pervasive disturbance in how the person experiences themselves, other people, and the world, which manifests in maladaptive patterns of thinking, emotional experience, emotional expression, and behaviour. Specifically, complex PTSD is characterised by a distorted view of the self (e.g., guilt, shame, and defeat), difficulties with intimacy in relationships, and affective dysregulation. This will inevitably resemble disturbances in aspects of the self (e.g., self-esteem) and disruption in interpersonal functioning (e.g., intimacy avoidance), which together can manifest as both over- and under-regulation of emotions. Many individuals with complex PTSD will therefore naturally fulfil the diagnostic requirements for a Personality Disorder.

Although both diagnoses can in fact be assigned simultaneously, ICD-11 stipulates that Personality Disorder must not be better explained by another disorder. If a patient with PTSD also has symptoms of distorted self-view, problems with intimacy, and emotion regulation and the onset of symptoms are directly related to an event or series of events of an extremely threatening or horrific nature, the diagnosis should generally be complex PTSD and not Personality Disorder. In some cases, however, it may make sense to make both diagnoses; for example, when the Personality Disorder diagnosis contributes relevant information that is not adequately covered by the complex PTSD diagnosis (e.g., incoherent and unstable self-view with fluctuations between unrealistically positive and negative self-perceptions) or is decidedly incompatible with complex PTSD (e.g., dominating or manipulative behaviour). This could, for example, be a patient with a highly unstable or grandiose self-perception, which is generally not attributable to complex PTSD. Both diagnoses should also be made in cases where substantial Personality Disorder features are likely to have been present prior to traumatisation (Felding et al., 2021). It is also important to emphasise that the duration requirement for complex PTSD is only "several weeks of symptoms," while for Personality Disorder it is "two years or more." The problems that characterise Personality Disorder are thus somewhat more habitual compared to complex PTSD.

To summarise, the clinician can use the rule of thumb that, if there are traumatic events (i.e., events of an extremely threatening or horrific nature) and clear PTSD core symptoms in the medical history, complex PTSD should generally be ruled out before diagnosing a Personality Disorder. At the same time, however, it should be noted that trauma is very common both in the general population and especially in psychiatric populations, which is why it is the core PTSD symptoms and their connection to trauma that are crucial for diagnosis. One of the key symptoms in the ICD-11 PTSD diagnosis is the re-experiencing symptom, which is quite a difficult symptom. It is not simply about being able to recall the trauma, but about involuntarily reliving the event or aspects of it in the present (Hyland et al., 2021). Finally, it is important to emphasise that the usefulness of diagnosing a concurrent Personality Disorder in such cases depends on the specific clinical situation (e.g., an available treatment programme for Personality Disorder but not for complex PTSD).

Secondary Personality Change

Personality is generally relatively stable over time. Similarly, Personality Disorder and Personality Difficulty are usually also relatively stable from early adulthood onwards. In contrast, a Secondary Personality Change may present after or concurrently with an organic condition that is deemed to be the direct pathophysiological cause of the change. This takes the form of new or altered personality characteristics that represent a change from the person's previous personality pattern (e.g., prominent apathy, aggressiveness, emotional lability, suspiciousness, paranoid delusions, and deficient inhibition). In order to diagnose Secondary Personality Change, it is crucial to identify the presence of an organic condition that could potentially explain the personality change and that there is a temporal relationship between the two phenomena.

A number of diseases and conditions of the nervous system can form the basis for personality change, including head trauma, stroke, Huntington's disease, epilepsy, Parkinson's disease, multiple sclerosis, neural infectious diseases, low metabolism, and autoimmune diseases such as systemic lupus erythematosus. If symptoms of impaired personality functioning are caused by such organic conditions, a Personality Disorder should not be diagnosed.

Attention Deficit Hyperactivity Disorder (ADHD)

As with Personality Disorder, individuals with ADHD often have psychosocial impairment (e.g., problems completing school and training and maintaining employment) and interpersonal problems (e.g., forgetting appointments and interrupting others when speaking), which are also linked to problems with emotion regulation (e.g., strong sense of justice and low frustration tolerance). When ADHD persists into adolescence and adulthood, it can be particularly difficult to distinguish it from a Personality Disorder with prominent trait domains such as Disinhibition in the form of irresponsibility, impulsivity, distractibility, and risk-taking behaviour, and Negative Affectivity in the form of increased sensitivity to negative stimuli and a tendency towards anxiety, anger, and self-blame. It is also important to emphasise that research suggests that ADHD can be a route or precursor to the development of Personality Disorder, where emotional dysregulation and psychosocial experiences of failure throughout childhood play a central role (Matthies & Philipsen, 2016; Storebø & Simonsen, 2014). The usefulness of diagnosing ADHD alongside a Personality Disorder generally also depends on the specific clinical situation.

Dissociative Identity Disorder

Moderate to Severe Personality Disorder may in some cases be characterised by dissociative states or symptoms that occur exclusively under stressful conditions. Such dissociative phenomena may include, for example, out-of-body experiences, sense of alienation, depersonalisation, and amnesia (e.g., not remembering what you said or did during an affect-related blackout). Similarly, people with a Dissociative or Partial Dissociative Identity Disorder may, for example, experience amnesia related to a certain behaviour as if they were a different person while performing certain actions. A disjointed sense of self and lack of purpose characterise both Dissociative Identity Disorder and many people with Personality Disorder. Furthermore, both Personality Disorder and Dissociative Identity Disorder are characterised by a tendency to have experienced trauma and stress throughout life. Particularly in Partial Dissociative Identity Disorder, there may be milder or shorter episodes of amnesia that are limited to extreme emotional states or self-harm, which can also result from Moderate to Severe Personality Disorder.

Thus, in both Dissociative Identity Disorder and Personality Disorder, there may be persistent difficulties with sense of identity, goal orientation, and emotion regulation. With respect to differential diagnosis, Personality Disorder does not involve two or more distinct personality states, but some individuals with Moderate to Severe Personality Disorder may have transient dissociative experiences in situations of stress or intense emotion.

Dysthymic Disorder

Dysthymic Disorder (also referred to as dysthymia) might be difficult to distinguish from Personality Disorder, which is partly due to the fact that it has traditionally been referred to as a Depressive Personality Disorder (Huprich, 2013). The diagnosis has a gradual onset in childhood, adolescence, or early adulthood, which already overlaps with Personality Disorder. Next, it is a condition or disorder that is relatively persistent, which for both dysthymia and Personality Disorder translates as "two years or more." Characteristic symptoms include persistent low self-esteem, negativity, and pessimism, which can also be core aspects of Personality Disorder (e.g., aspects of the self and the trait domain of Negative Affectivity). Finally, dysthymia often co-occurs with other mental disorders, such as anxiety disorders, OCD, addictions, and eating disorders, which is also very much the case for Personality Disorder. However, this is where the commonalities seem to end. The depressive mood should generally only last most of the day or most days in the form of feeling sad or "down." From the outside, the person may appear tearful and characterised by a sense of defeat. In children and adolescents, these dysthymic characteristics can sometimes manifest as all-encompassing irritability. There is a considerable incidence of concurrent dysthymia and Personality Disorder, probably representing what used to be called Depressive Personality Disorder.

Separation Anxiety Disorder

Separation Anxiety Disorder is characterised by a pronounced and excessive fear or anxiety of separation from specific attachment figures. Most people associate this disorder with children and adolescents, where the anxiety is typically orientated towards parents or other caregivers. However, Separation Anxiety is just as common among adults, where symptoms are typically linked to a partner or their own children. It is well known that abandonment anxiety and interpersonal dependency on others can also be manifestations of a Personality Disorder but, in Personality Disorder, these symptoms are usually accompanied by problems with interpersonal functioning, emotion regulation, and identity boundaries. Personality Disorder and Separation Anxiety can be diagnosed simultaneously but, as a general rule, Separation Anxiety should not be diagnosed if the symptoms are best explained by Personality Disorder. Finally, Separation Anxiety Disorder must have been present for at least "several months," while Personality Disorder must have been present for "two years or more."

Social Anxiety Disorder

Social Anxiety Disorder is characterised by marked and excessive fear or anxiety that consistently occur in one or more social situations such as social interactions (e.g., having a conversation), doing something while feeling observed (e.g., eating or drinking in the presence of others), or performing in front of others (e.g., giving a speech). The individual is typically concerned that they will act in a way, or present with visible anxiety symptoms, that will be negatively evaluated by others. Such anxiousness and social concerns may resemble what is often seen in personality disordered individuals with prominent traits of Negative Affectivity (e.g., social anxiousness) and Detachment (e.g., social withdrawal). The concern about being negatively evaluated by others may resemble compromised perspective-taking where the individual reads too much in between the lines of what other people think, say, and do (i.e., hyper-mentalisation). Moreover, both disorders may also be characterised by inaccurate situational and interpersonal appraisals under stress, which for both may lead to distortions (e.g., "everyone stares at me and think I am stupid because of what I just said").

For both Social Anxiety Disorder and Personality Disorder, the symptoms must not be transient but should persist for an extended period. ICD-11 explicitly states that Social Anxiety Disorder is generally considered to be a chronic condition, which is also comparable to a Personality Disorder. However, symptoms of Social Anxiety Disorder must only persist for at least several months, while a Personality Disorder must persist around 2 years or more.

Similar to a Personality Disorder, the onset of Social Anxiety Disorder typically occurs during childhood and adolescence, with a large majority of cases emerging between 8 and 15 years of age.

This gradual emergence of Social Anxiety Disorder may easily be confused with Personality Disorder, which also emerges in the process of personality development during these years. But, in some cases, Social Anxiety Disorder occurs precipitously subsequent to a stressful or humiliating social experience (e.g., school bullying), which is unlikely for a Personality Disorder where more pervasive early adversity is often the case (e.g., emotional abuse and neglect by parental figures).

In cases where Social Anxiety Disorder is strongly generalised to many situations and settings (i.e., being pervasive), it may be more challenging to differentiate it from a Personality Disorder, which is pervasive by nature. However, in many cases, Social Anxiety Disorders occurs in fairly specific situations (e.g., with authorities, the opposite sex, talking in front of the class), which is less pervasive than what is typically seen in Personality Disorder where aspects of social inhibition may not only apply to peers and authorities but also or especially in the most intimate relationships (e.g., finding it hard to be open with people they are close to).

Obsessive-Compulsive Disorder (OCD)

OCD often characterises the clinical picture of a person over a long period of time and sometimes to such a degree that it is best described as being pervasive, including high Conscientiousness. Similarly, Personality Disorder can be characterised by Anankastia, which includes a maladaptive pattern of excessive perfectionism and rigid control. In terms of differential diagnosis, it is important to emphasise that individuals with this Personality Disorder do not necessarily experience the OCD-specific intrusive thoughts, images, impulses, or urges that can also manifest as recurrent patterns of obsessions or compulsions. In people with OCD, the symptoms will generally be unwanted and distressing, similar to what is traditionally referred to as *ego-dystonia*. In contrast, a Personality Disorder with prominent anankastic traits will usually involve a perfectionistic and rigid approach to oneself and other people that the person has no desire to change and can therefore be considered *ego-syntonic*. Basically, if the requirements for both OCD and a Personality Disorder are met, both diagnoses can be made.

Conduct-Dissocial Disorder

Conduct-Dissocial Disorder is a diagnosis that can only be made in children and adolescents, potentially overlapping with Personality Disorder, which can also be diagnosed in minors. Conduct-Dissocial Disorder is characterised by a recurrent pattern of behaviour that violates the basic rights of others and age-appropriate social or cultural norms, rules, or laws. The diagnosis can occur for a limited period of time, lasting a year or so, but can also be lifelong.

Although the disorder is very much related to the characteristics of a Personality Disorder with prominent Dissociality and Disinhibition, it is not an actual Personality Disorder. However, there is probably no significant difference between the two diagnoses, other than that Conduct-Dissocial Disorder can only be diagnosed in children and adolescents, even before the teenage years, which is generally not possible with Personality Disorder. In order to diagnose Conduct-Dissocial Disorder, the pattern must have lasted approximately 1 year or more. In comparison, a Personality Disorder generally needs to have lasted about 2 years or more, which is a full year more. In practice, it can often be difficult to precisely assess such duration requirements when it comes to diagnosis with childhood onset.

Among individuals with Conduct-Dissocial Disorder, an additional diagnosis of Personality Disorder is only warranted if there are personality features in addition to Dissociality (e.g., Negative Affectivity and Detachment) that contribute to significant impairments in aspects of the self or problems with interpersonal functioning.

Disorders Due to Substance Use or Addictive Behaviours

Here, we highlight differential diagnostic considerations in relation to addiction problems, including addiction to drugs, gambling, and video games.

Disorders attributed to substance use often have a profound impact on self and interpersonal functioning. For example, substance abuse can lead to problems with goal-directedness (e.g., preventing savings due to drug spending), conflicts in relationships (e.g., taking advantage of others' financial resources and being cut off from one's social network), dissocial behaviour (e.g., deceptive, manipulative, or violent) related to obtaining or using drugs, as well as a host of other characteristics often seen in individuals with a Personality Disorder.

If the personality problems are solely due to substance abuse, it should not lead to a diagnosis of Personality Disorder. However, if the personality problems in question cannot be fully explained by substance abuse (e.g., if the personality pattern precedes the substance abuse), or if characteristics of a Personality Disorder are seen that cannot be solely attributed to substance use (e.g., excessive perfectionism), a concurrent diagnosis of Personality Disorder may be warranted. Overall, it is important to consider that a majority of drug abusers are likely to have an underlying Personality Disorder or, conversely, that many people with a Personality Disorder can be expected to have a Disorder Due to Substance Use (Verheul, 2001). This natural correlation is partly due to the fact that drugs can act as a soothing or stimulating coping strategy for difficult emotions or situations. Here, there can often be a correlation between prominent trait domains and type of substance abuse. For example, individuals with prominent Dissociality may be inclined to use cocaine in order to further boost their own grandiosity and dominance (Weiss & Mirin, 1986).

In addition to drug addiction, people with Personality Disorder may also be prone to developing an addiction to gambling, also known as compulsive gambling. This is especially true in Personality Disorders with prominent Disinhibition (e.g., impulsivity and risk-taking behaviour). Therefore, ICD-11 allows for gambling addiction to be diagnosed alongside a Personality Disorder when appropriate. By extension, it should be mentioned that, in many cases, gambling addiction could also be associated with underlying personality disturbances. In cases where addictions co-occur with Personality Disorder, the most prominent trait domains are typically Negative Affectivity and Disinhibition (Müller et al., 2023).

Impulse Control Disorders

Here, we will highlight considerations of differential diagnoses in terms of impulse control disorders, including Intermittent Explosive Disorder, Compulsive Sexual Behaviour Disorder, Pyromania, and Kleptomania. Intermittent Explosive Disorder involves a pattern of recurrent, transient explosive episodes involving verbal (e.g., verbal attack on another person, rage outbursts, yelling) or physical aggression by an individual. Some individuals with Intermittent Explosive Disorder are likely to meet the diagnostic requirements for a Personality Disorder with prominent Disinhibition (e.g., impulsivity and risk-taking behaviour) and Negative Affectivity (e.g., low frustration tolerance, overreactive emotionality, anger, and hostility). However, Intermittent Explosive Disorder only needs to occur regularly over a period of 3 months or at a lower frequency over the course of a year if the outbursts are more intense. In comparison, the duration of a Personality Disorder should be approximately 2 years or more, usually with onset in adolescence. The aggressive behaviour must not be attributable to instrumental dissocial behaviour as in a Personality Disorder with prominent Dissociality, and the outbursts must not be considered beneficial to the person (Sellbom et al., 2018). It only makes sense to diagnose a concurrent Personality Disorder if there are pervasive and persistent problems with self and interpersonal functioning that go beyond what can be explained by an Intermittent Explosive Disorder alone. Overall, both diagnoses can be made if all diagnostic requirements are met for each. The utility of further diagnosing a Personality Disorder in this case depends on the specific clinical situation.

Another diagnosis that can be confused or co-exist with Personality Disorder in some cases is Compulsive Sexual Behaviour Disorder. For example, some people with Personality Disorder may engage in recurrent sexual behaviour as a dysfunctional or destructive self-regulation strategy (e.g., to soothe or reduce the pressure of emotional distress or to stabilise self-esteem). Although both diagnoses can be made simultaneously, an additional diagnosis of Compulsive Sexual Behaviour Disorder is not warranted if the sexual behaviour is solely due to emotional dysregulation such as sexual self-harm, self-victimisation, or other coping strategies and characteristics of Personality Disorder.

As for the destructive behaviour associated with Pyromania, people with Personality Disorder may also engage in arson as part of a more pervasive pattern of dissocial behaviour, often for instrumental purposes (self-gain or revenge). In the case of Pyromania, arson will only be used to release a tension or accumulated affect. In general, people diagnosed with Pyromania do not exhibit any other dissocial behaviour than the arson itself. Similarly, the theft behaviour of Kleptomania can also occur in people with Personality Disorder and prominent Dissociality, where theft can be part of the overall symptom picture. It should also be noted that people with Kleptomania only do not exhibit dissocial behaviour other than the theft itself. However, it is not unusual for Pyromania and Kleptomania to be diagnosed along with a Personality Disorder.

Manifestations and Development From Childhood to Old Age

There is a tendency for personality disturbances to first manifest themselves during childhood, increasing in intensity through early adolescence, and continuing to grow from adolescence into adulthood, although symptoms may not come into clinical attention until later in life. Clinicians are generally advised to be cautious about diagnosing Personality Disorder too early because children's personalities are still developing. Conversely, it is also not appropriate to avoid early detection and treatment (Chanen & McCutcheon, 2008; Kongerslev et al., 2015). This poses a clinical dilemma that in each case ultimately depends on sound clinical judgement.

Developmental Aspects of Personality Functioning

Personality Disorder is not commonly diagnosed in children before puberty. During the course of their development, children gain knowledge and experiences about themselves and other people, which are integrated into a coherent identity and self-understanding as well as individual ways of interacting with others. As there are significant differences in how this maturation process occurs, it can be difficult to determine whether a prepubertal child shows signs of disturbance in aspects of the self (e.g., identity, self-esteem, and accuracy of self-view) because these functions are not yet fully developed. This also applies to interpersonal functioning (e.g., the ability to understand other people's perspectives and managing conflict in relationships).

When assessing teenagers, it is important to consider normative manifestations in this age group. For example, mood swings, risk-taking behaviour, and self-harm are more common in adolescence than in adulthood. Aspects of identity and social roles are also known to be more experimental and changeable in teenagers than what is commonly seen in adults. Therefore, the diagnostic threshold for whether such patterns are indicative of

Personality Disorder should also be higher in teenagers. Furthermore, the clinician should consider the wide variation in what is considered normal development in teenagers (e.g., moodiness, irritability, and social insecurity).

In this context, it should be emphasised that ICD-11 describes Personality Disorder as a *relatively* stable diagnosis that typically emerges in early adulthood. The term "relative" indicates that the disorder can change over time, so that a person diagnosed in early adulthood no longer fulfils the diagnostic requirements in middle age. More unusually, a person who previously did not have a diagnosable Personality Disorder (e.g., due to adequate psychosocial functioning) may develop one later in life. The question here is whether this is a late onset development or manifestation of the Personality Disorder? When a Personality Disorder manifests in older adults, according to ICD-11, it may be associated with a loss of social support that previously helped the person to compensate for personality difficulties and thereby maintain adequate psychosocial functioning. When personality change occurs in middle-aged or older adults without a change in their life circumstances, it is especially important to assess whether the change may be due to an underlying medical condition (i.e., Secondary Personality Change) or an undetected disorder due to substance use.

Trait Domains in Children Versus Adults

Prominent maladaptive traits are often observable in pre-teens and constitute true precursors to trait expressions of a Personality Disorder in adolescence and adulthood. For example, trait domains such as Negative Affectivity and Disinhibition as well as more specific facets such as lack of empathy (facet under Dissociality) and perfectionism (facet under Anankastia) can be observed in very young children. However, such traits are also associated with the development of other mental disorders (e.g., affective and anxiety based) and should therefore not automatically be interpreted as clear early manifestations of Personality Disorder.

Generally, behavioural expressions of Dissociality and Disinhibition tend to decline over the course of adulthood, so that older individuals will typically be more altruistic, kind, indulgent, and conscientious than teenagers. On the other hand, trait domains such as Detachment and Anankastia tend to decrease only slightly over time. If you have an introverted nature, as is often the case with Detachment, you will usually remain introverted for the rest of your life. Similarly, children and adolescents with predominant Anankastia will usually continue to make high demands on themselves and others, even as they get older.

Given the aforementioned developmental manifestations of trait domains, it is important to consider the implications for a clinical diagnosis. We know that levels of Disinhibition (e.g., risk-taking behaviour) and Negative Affectivity (e.g., emotional reactions that are out of proportion) are naturally higher in teenagers and adolescents than in adults. Therefore, the threshold for determining whether these trait domains contribute to a Personality Disorder diagnosis should also be correspondingly higher.

Personality Disorder and Other Co-Occurring Mental Disorders

With ICD-11 it is definitively clarified that it is in fact possible to assign multiple concurrent diagnoses, and that it is predominantly a clinical judgement whether it makes sense to add the diagnosis of Personality Disorder for a person who, for example, also has a diagnosis of PTSD or Schizophrenia. It is also important that ICD-11 now only uses the term "comorbidity" in cases where there is a concurrent somatic or organic disorder. In other words, when there are two or more mental disorders, which occur simultaneously, they are simply co-occurring disorders. This is because the concept of comorbidity assumes that two or more conditions can be distinguished from each other; for example, based on cause or processes of biological disease. The working group behind the ICD-11 classification has repeatedly pointed out that the categorical diagnosis of Personality Disorders has contributed to problematic underdiagnosis in clinical practice (Pedersen & Simonsen, 2014; Tyrer et al., 2015). Presumably, in most cases, this underdiagnosis is due to clinicians failing to diagnose personality disorders when there is a co-occurring and treatment-requiring anxiety, depression, or eating disorder. Studies suggest that more than one in 10 people in the general population (Volkert et al., 2018) and 50–80% of patients in outpatient psychiatric treatment have a Personality Disorder (Alnæs & Torgersen, 1988; Beckwith et al., 2014). Whether or not a Personality Disorder is diagnosed can have consequences for the extent and type of treatment and for the understanding of the overall symptom pattern. In addition, a significant advantage of adding a concurrent Personality Disorder diagnosis is that the clinician thereby supports a psychological framework or context for the person's disorder that is not provided by talking about, for example, a diagnosis of anxiety or depression (Swales, 2022; Tyrer et al., 2022). In this way, the linking of personality concepts to a person's disorder can be seen as an aspect of clinical applicability, which we will return to in Chapter 6.

Three general models can be described to understand the relationship between Personality Disorder and other mental disorders, which are discussed in the next three sections (Widiger, 2011).

Non-Causal Pathoplasticity

Non-causal pathoplasticity occurs in cases where two disorders are present, and one disorder affects the presentation or expression of the other disorder. An example would be the relationship between a Personality Disorder with predominant Anankastia (e.g., perfectionism) and anorectic Eating Disorder. Although perfectionism is not the cause of Anorexia Nervosa, perfectionism can have a significant impact on how anorexia is expressed (Lavender et al., 2013). Another example could be the presence of somatic illness in a person with personality disturbances characterised by Negative Affectivity, where the latter will naturally affect the person's ability to cope with their somatic disorder (Goodwin et al., 2006; Widiger & Oltmanns, 2017).

Shared Aetiology on the Same Spectrum

Although in most cases we do not know the specific aetiology behind mental disorders, there are several examples of disorders where we know of common factors that cut across the disorders. These can be both biological and psychosocial factors that help explain symptoms, which can then be said to be within the same spectrum. Examples of this could be the relationship between prevalent Negative Affectivity (e.g., anxiousness) and Detachment (e.g., social avoidance) on the one hand and social phobia on the other. It can also manifest as a continuum between predominant Anankastia and OCD.

Bidirectional Causal Impact

Bidirectional causal influence occurs in cases where two different diagnoses are present and causally influence each other. A common clinical example of this could be the relationship between predominant Negative Affectivity on the one hand and depression on the other, where we know that distinct episodes of depression are often present early in life in people with prominent Negative Affectivity, which may also influence its trait intensity, but also that Negative Affectivity itself is predisposing to depressive episodes.

There is no test or study that can be used to verify which of the three models is relevant to the individual case. Nevertheless, we believe that a theoretical understanding can be both practical (e.g., in relation to treatment planning) and contribute to a more humane and personality-grounded understanding of the many patients who experience inadequate treatment in often very limited programmes. Based on quite extensive evidence, ICD-11 points out that Personality Disorder both complicates and often requires prolonged treatment of concurrent clinical syndromes such as anxiety and depression (Newton-Howes et al., 2014; Tyrer et al., 2022). In many cases, an inadequate response to standard treatment can thus indicate the presence of a Personality Disorder.

Dimensions Are Coded as Categories

The ICD-11 classification we describe has typically been referred to as a "dimensional" approach, emphasising a continuum between adaptive and maladaptive characteristics. This focus on dimensions has raised concerns among some clinicians, who favour more definitive categories to facilitate clinical decision making, planning, and targeted treatment. It is perhaps important to note that while both severity and trait domains have a dimensional nature, the diagnostic codes can really only be used as categories. Thus, Personality Disorder severity can only be classified based on three categories, while trait domains are categorically either assigned or not assigned.

A general practitioner or other healthcare professionals must first and foremost decide whether the patient has a Personality Disorder based on the general diagnostic requirements, which is essentially a categorical decision. Subsequently, the clinician must decide whether the patient has a Mild, Moderate, or Severe Personality Disorder, which is also a categorical decision. This is similar to diagnosing a Depressive Episode, which can also be specified as a Mild, Moderate, or Severe Depressive Episode. Next, the most prominent trait domains are recorded, which are also only coded as present or absent, even though they actually exist on a continuum. So, are we dealing with dimensions or categories? The answer is essentially both. From a scientific perspective, we are dealing with dimensions (e.g., there is no definitively true threshold between "mild" and "moderate"), but in clinical practice, there is no other option but to code the dimensions as categories. These two different perspectives offer different possibilities. On the one hand, clinical psychologists can draw dimensional portraits of the patient's difficulties (and resources), where both low and high scores, including sub-diagnostic levels, are included in the interpretation. On the other hand, practitioners can translate the profile into diagnostic categories for clinical decision making. Eventually, it will also make sense to convert a dimensional "measurement" of severity into diagnostic severity categories using norm-based thresholds or other relevant markers (Bach et al., 2023). Such diagnostic categorisations will be empirically substantiated, unlike the previous categories.

After all, dimensions are not all that foreign in healthcare. For example, it is common for physicians to work with a continuum of bone density in all people, where a certain low level ("cut-off") is used to diagnose the condition osteoporosis. The same applies to the body mass index dimension, which is used to diagnose Anorexia Nervosa and other eating disorders. The key point is that everyone can have different levels of bone density and body mass index without necessarily being diagnosed.

Chapter 3

Clinical Understanding of Personality Functioning

With this chapter we will introduce the reader to the most important aspects of personality functioning, which is a prerequisite for diagnosing and determining the severity of a Personality Disorder described more specifically in Chapter 4. The starting point is the crucial information on capacities and manifestations presented in Box 3.1.

Gordon Allport writes in his definition of personality: "Personality *is* something and *does* something. It is not synonymous with behaviour or activity, least of all it is merely the impression that this activity makes on others. It is what lies *behind* specific acts and *within the* individual" (Allport, 1937, p. 48). According to Allport, when we talk about a person's personality, we can focus on what the personality *is* (e.g., tendency to be withdrawn, anxious, perfectionistic, or callous) and what the personality *does* (e.g., makes plans and realises them, empathises with others, and shares life with them). It is particularly the latter aspects of personality that ICD-11 emphasises when diagnosing the global severity of a Personality Disorder (mild, moderate, severe). Determining the severity is the primary part of the classification, as this assessment determines whether behaviours or symptoms fall within the category of Personality Disorder at all and, by extension, can be treated (e.g., with different levels of treatment intensity). Overall, Personality Disorder is defined in ICD-11 as a disturbance in aspects of the self and interpersonal functioning, that is, one's relationship with oneself and with other people. Thus, to determine whether a Personality Disorder is mild, moderate, or severe, we consider the degree of problems in the person's relationship with themself and other people along with the degree of emotional, cognitive, and behavioural manifestations of these problems. Last, but not least, a global assessment of psychosocial impairment and distress is fundamental to diagnosing severity. In this regard, note that there is usually a close correlation between the different capacities of personality functioning, even though they are described in Box 3.1 as relatively distinct. The skilled clinician will be able to recognise and articulate connections between the different capacities and manifestations in ways that are interpenetrating and add psychological coherence and meaning.

Box 3.1.

Aspects of personality functioning that contribute to severity determination in Personality Disorder

- Degree and pervasiveness of disturbances in functioning of aspects of the self:
  - Stability and coherence of one's sense of identity (e.g., extent to which identity or sense of self is variable and inconsistent or overly rigid and fixed)
  - Ability to maintain an overall positive and stable sense of self-worth
  - Accuracy of one's view of one's characteristics, strengths, limitations
  - Capacity for self-direction (ability to plan, choose, and implement appropriate goals)
- Degree and pervasiveness of interpersonal dysfunction across various contexts and relationships (e.g., romantic relationships, school/work, parent–child, family, friendships, peer contexts):
  - Interest in engaging in relationships with others
  - Ability to understand and appreciate others' perspectives
  - Ability to develop and maintain close and mutually satisfying relationships
  - Ability to manage conflict in relationships
- Pervasiveness, severity, and chronicity of emotional, cognitive, and behavioural manifestations of the personality dysfunction:
  Emotional manifestations:
  - Range and appropriateness of emotional experience and expression
  - Tendency to be emotionally over- or underreactive
  - Ability to recognise and acknowledge emotions that are difficult or unwanted by the individual (e.g., anger, sadness)
  Cognitive manifestations:
  - Accuracy of situational and interpersonal appraisals, especially under stress
  - Ability to make appropriate decisions in situations of uncertainty
  - Appropriate stability and flexibility of belief systems
  Behavioural manifestations:
  - Flexibility in controlling impulses and modulating behaviour based on the situation and consideration of the consequences
  - Appropriateness of behavioural responses to intense emotions and stressful circumstances (e.g., propensity to self-harm or violence)
- The extent to which the dysfunctions in the above areas are associated with distress or impairment in personal, family, social, educational, occupational, or other important areas of functioning.

(World Health Organization, 2024, p. 555)

Aspects of the Self

The following defines and exemplifies the four capacities related to aspects of the self: identity, self-esteem, self-view, and self-direction. These capacities are naturally intertwined with each other (e.g., self-worth is associated with self-view) and interact with aspects of interpersonal functioning (e.g., low self-esteem often contributes to a negative perception of how one is viewed by others). Examples of functional and dysfunctional aspects of the self are shown in Table 3.1.

Table 3.1   Examples of adaptive and maladaptive aspects of the self

Adaptive functioning	Maladaptive functioning
Stability and coherence in sense of identity ("has a common thread")	Lacking a sense of coherent and stable identity ("missing the common thread")
Ability to maintain an overall positive and stable sense of self-worth	Dysregulated self-esteem – either pronounced inferiority or grandiose self-perception
Accuracy in recognising own attributes, strengths, and limitations	Feelings of inadequacy causing social avoidance Self-perception marked by overconfidence Mismatch between skills and actions
Ability to plan, select, and implement appropriate goals	Confusion or lack of agency and self-direction Goal inhibition, procrastination, risk aversion Overly or rigidly goal orientated

Identity

In a healthy personality, the identity is usually stable and coherent, meaning a consistent sense of self and a well-integrated interaction between different aspects of the person. Such capacity enables us to determine what is important and valuable to us, make appropriate plans and stick to them, and organize our lives accordingly (Taylor, 1989; Lind et al., 2020). In personality dysfunction, there will either be significant variation, instability, or contradictions in self-view and identity ("missing the common thread"), or identity and self-view may be overly rigid and fixed. For the philosophically interested reader, Paul Ricoeur (1992) distinguishes between the stable and permanent components of the self ("idem") and the more adaptable, changing, and dynamic aspects of the self ("ipse"). A healthy narrative identity constructively balances between these two poles. In this respect, identity dysfunction can be said to be characterised by the ipse being deprived of support from the idem, meaning that the changing aspects of the ipse are not integrated with the more stable and permanent aspects of the idem. On the one hand, this can result in an overly stable or rigid identity while on the other hand, it may result in an overly flexible and disjointed identity.

From a developmental psychopathology perspective, both positive and negative experiences from childhood ("inner models") are sought to be integrated and organised into a coherent whole (Caligor et al., 2018; Hörz-Sagstetter et al., 2021). When this integration does not take place in an adequate way, it can lead to identity disturbances, which can be reflected in an overly inflexible and rigid identity or an overly flexible and incoherent identity (Blüml & Doering, 2021; Fonagy & Target, 2003; Jørgensen et al., 2024). As shown in Figure 3.1, an optimal identity functioning will accommodate the capacity to be flexible while maintaining a fixed and well-defined identity that corresponds to a sense of personal integrity and appropriate adaptability in life.

Most of us have an experience of a core self but, at the same time, we should be able to flexibly adjust and adapt our sense of identity and self-presentation to changes in surroundings and circumstances (e.g., appearing competent and professional at a job interview, while also allowing a more sensitive, authentic, and relaxed side at home on the couch). In this way, we are like diamonds that, depending on the context, can bring out a certain side that best suits the

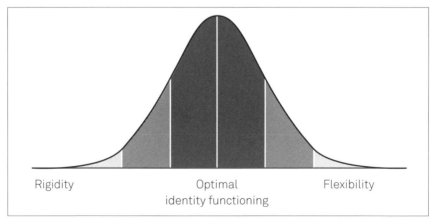

Rigidity   Optimal   Flexibility
                      identity functioning

Figure 3.1 Identity functioning where extreme rigidity and extreme flexibility represent opposite poles of the spectrum

context without compromising the person we really are. If the identity is too incoherent, then even slight pressure or stress may cause the person to become emotionally overwhelmed, causing the identity to dissolve or merge with the identity of others. On the other hand, if the identity is too fixed or rigid, this can also cause problems in both self-perception and in relationships (e.g., difficulty letting go of the professional side of the identity and surrendering to the relaxed side at home on the couch). In other words, this is a matter of experiencing and living out one's identity in an authentic and flexible manner and not only experience and live out the fixed identity one may have been given by talent, education, skills, or position. Sometimes people's talents can take them beyond their character, meaning that certain people only experience and live out who they are on the outside (e.g., their professional uniform) and not who they are on the inside (e.g., a parent, spouse, friend).

An optimal identity functioning can be compared to a diamond, which has a stable core while still having many different sides to show off. Following the same metaphor, an inflexible and rigid identity can be compared to a squared stone where all sides are the same, while an overly flexible and disjointed identity corresponds to an intangible and boundless substance or a stone that is fragmented beyond recognition.

- In *dialectical behavioural therapy,* Identity Disorder is understood as an expression of dysfunctional self-regulation, which includes not only emotions and behaviour, but also feelings of emptiness and difficulty understanding oneself. In therapy, this is addressed by working with goals and values in life and a general dialectical focus on integrating opposing aspects of the self through synthesis and acceptance (Linehan, 1993).
- In *mentalisation-based therapy,* Identity Disorder is understood as an expression of a compromised ability to mentalise (i.e., the ability to process and understand mental states of oneself and others). People with identity problems often express a sense of confusion about whether thoughts and emotions belong to themselves or to others. In therapy, this is addressed by working with and strengthening the ability to mentalise, thereby increasing self-understanding and inner coherence (Bateman & Fonagy, 2016).
- In *schema therapy,* Identity Disorder is understood, among other things, as an expression of enduring shifts between activated and disintegrated self-schemas and coping responses ("modes"), each reflecting a different view of the self. The greater the severity of the Personality Disorder, the more dominant and disintegrated these modes are. In addition, a highly over-compliant "mode" can compromise the person's ability to develop an independent healthy adult identity, because they instead accommodate and adopt the attitudes, preferences, and interests of others (Young et al., 2003).

Identity disturbances are perceived by many as the most fundamental aspect of personality dysfunction, meaning that identity problems are related to virtually all of the other capacities and manifestations described in this chapter. Identity can be considered the central psychological structure that organises a person's experience of self (and thereby also their experience of others). This self-organisation includes a unified sense of self in relation to the world, which is continuously activated by inner models of self and others. Inner mental models include the building blocks that need to be integrated to form a coherent identity and sense of self. Fundamentally, the level of identity consolidation or cohesiveness distinguishes a healthy level of personality functioning from disturbed levels of personality functioning (Caligor et al., 2018; Jørgensen et al., 2024). Healthy identity functioning involves an integrated sense of self that is complex, realistic, and continuous across time and situation. This manifests as an ability to maintain engagement in intellectual, professional, and recreational interests, and to know one's own mind in terms of values, opinions, beliefs, and tastes. This coherent identity plays a central role in the other capacities of personality functioning, such as healthy self-esteem, interpersonal engagement, adaptive decision making, pursuit of long-term goals, and experience and tolerance of negative affect without compromised impulse control or reality testing. The most severe Personality Disorders are characterised by the use of immature coping strategies or defense mechanisms such as splitting and dissociation that create a fragmented identity. Over the long run this perpetuates unstable, distorted, superficial, and/or emotionally abnormal experiences of self and others. In addition, the ability to identify and pursue long-term goals is often impaired, while relationships with others become avoidant, unstable, superficial, and exploitative or based solely on the fulfilment of immediate needs. Many people with Severe Personality Disorder struggle with not being able to tolerate being alone and needing the constant presence of another person, while their fragmented experience of self and others creates an equally unbearable dynamic when in a relationship.

> In summary, identity can be seen as a central psychological structure that organises a person's perception of themselves and, in turn, their perception of others. Identity problems are therefore often most evident in social contexts. Healthy identity functioning implies an integrated sense of self that is complex, realistic, and continuous across time and situations, which is essential for all personality capacities and manifestations, including:
> - Knowing your own mind in terms of values, opinions, beliefs, and tastes
> - A healthy self-esteem
> - Experiencing and tolerating negative affect without impaired impulse control or reality testing
> - Ability to work and collaborate
> - Pursuit of long-term goals including intellectual, recreational, and professional interests

It might be important to distinguish between the person's narrative or autobiographical self and the more pervasive core self (Zandersen & Parnas, 2018). This distinction can in many ways be equated with William James's definitions of "knower" and "known" (Jørgensen, 2006). When the core self is disturbed (so-called self-disorder or anomalous self-experience), it can include persistent and often agonising experiences of not being able to feel yourself or figure out who you are. In schizophrenia spectrum disorders, this is more enduring and not situationally anchored. People with Severe Personality Disorder may also experience a lack of sense of self, but this will often alternate between a lack of sense of self and very intense self-experiences (i.e., contradictory sense of self). In contrast to people with Schizophrenia, such interactions can often be linked to situational or relational triggers in people with Personality Disorders It may therefore be necessary for clinicians to spend extra time investigating identity functioning in order to rule out possible self-disorder as present in Schizophrenia.

Examples of identity issues in internalising versus externalising problems

Individuals with *internalising* problems (e.g., Negative Affectivity and Detachment) will often have an excessive tendency to submit to and seek recognition from other people in order to define their own place in this world (e.g., a sense of being supported and accepted) at the expense of healthy and independent identity formation. Similarly, individuals with *externalising* problems (e.g., Dissociality and Disinhibition) may exhibit excessive craving for the attention, respect, and admiration of others in order to increase their sense of importance (e.g., grandiose attention seeking). They may also have a rigid sense of identity due to their sense of entitlement or belief that they are special and therefore deserve certain benefits, relationships, or positions. For example, their ambitions and perceived talents may take them beyond who they actually are.

If you as a clinician want to uncover these characteristics in the patient, you can get started by asking, for example, "How would you describe yourself?" and "What kind of person are you?" and at the same time use your clinical observation of the extent to which the person has a clear sense of self even under stress. Here, it will often work best to start with a specific stressful situation and then ask closely about the experience of self and others. If the person is able to give realistic and coherent descriptions, this indicates a more well-functioning personality. Conversely, poor or unrealistic descriptions may indicate more severe identity dysfunction (see Table 3.2).

Table 3.2   Examples of severity levels of disrupted identity

Mild	The sense of self can be somewhat contradictory and not in line with how others see them
Moderate	Self-awareness can become decidedly incoherent during experienced crises
Severe	Self-view is highly unrealistic and typically very unstable or contradictory

Self-Esteem

In a healthy personality, there will be a solid ability to maintain an overall positive and stable sense of self-worth. Healthy self-esteem regulation involves neither an unrealistically low sense of self-worth (e.g., self-hatred) nor an unrealistically high sense of self-worth (e.g., grandiosity). For a Personality Disorder, there might be a consistently low self-esteem, a tendency to easily feel inferior, or a tendency for the self-esteem to be highly susceptible to circumstances (e.g., Caligor et al., 2018). In more complex or severe cases, there can be a shift between deflated and inflated sense of self-esteem, and sometimes even a complex, disintegrated, contradictory, and distressing combination of both aspects simultaneously (see Table 3.3).

Examples of self-esteem issues in internalising versus externalising problems

Individuals with *internalising* problems (e.g., Negative Affectivity and Detachment) can typically suffer from chronically low and unstable self-esteem, which can manifest as self-hatred and feelings of social inferiority. Individuals with *externalising* problems (e.g., Dissociality and Disinhibition) regulate their self-esteem using strategies that pose a risk to themselves and others, characteristically involving the use of power and acting out of personal gain at the expense of others. Externalising problems can also be associated with being overly self-confident and having self-aggrandising attitudes (e.g., inflated self-esteem with feelings of entitlement and special status).

If a clinician wants to uncover these characteristics in the patient, they can start by asking, for example, "How satisfied are you with yourself?" or "What gives you a sense of self-worth?" The clinician not only listens to the content of the answer, but also uses their clinical judgement in assessing the way these questions are answered and whether the life story provides credible examples of satisfying situations and relationships.

Table 3.3   Examples of severity levels of disordered self-esteem

Mild	Have difficulty recovering from experiences, where self-esteem has been injured (e.g., a slightly embarrassing situation)
Moderate	Have significant problems maintaining a positive self-esteem or have an unrealistically positive view of themselves
Severe	Have severe self-esteem regulation issues and self-esteem is often unstable or contradictory

View of Own Characteristics and Abilities

Identity and self-esteem are closely linked to the ability to take a relatively accurate view of one's own characteristics, strengths, and limitations. A healthy functioning person will usually have a realistic view of their own abilities, strengths, and limitations, while a person with personality dysfunction typically has an inaccurate or skewed view of such features. This is evidenced in research showing that the discrepancies between self and informant ratings of personality features increase as general personality pathology severity increases (Carnovale et al., 2019).

On the one hand, individuals with personality dysfunction may have a tendency to be overconfident, overestimate their abilities, and take risks even though they do not have the necessary abilities and resources. On the other hand, there may be a marked sense of inadequacy with an underestimation of their own abilities and characteristics, even though the person actually has the necessary characteristics and abilities to deal with the situation or task in question. Think of an anxious student who feels academically inferior to everyone else in their class, despite having good skills and insight into the material. Occasionally a complex mix of both over- and underestimation of one's own abilities can be seen in the same person, sometimes over time and sometimes simultaneously. There may also be a "mismatch" between abilities and actions, which can be attributed to neither over- nor underestimation of one's abilities, but rather should be seen as an expression of disintegrated identity.

Examples of self-view in internalising versus externalising problems

Individuals with *internalising* problems (e.g., Negative Affectivity and Detachment) may tend to underestimate their strengths and resources while overestimating their weaknesses and deficits. Similarly, people with *externalising* problems (e.g., Dissociality and Disinhibition) may tend to underestimate their own weaknesses and deficits while overestimating their own strengths and resources.

If clinicians want to uncover these traits in patients, one way to get started is to simply ask about the person's dreams and plans and compare them to the abilities and characteristics they possess.

Self-Direction

The capacity to act intentionally and be guided by a purpose is important for getting ahead in life and fulfilling life goals. It relies on a coherent sense of self in terms of knowing what is important, valuable, and true, which enables the person to set meaningful goals, stick to their goals, and eventually realize their goals (Taylor, 1989; Lind et al., 2020). Thus, goal-direction involves the ability to select, set, pursue, and realise appropriate and/or meaningful goals in life. This is a capacity that is closely linked to the human ability to construct a personal narrative of future goals, providing a sense of coherence and meaning that continuously supports and structures the person's goal and task orientation (Lind et al., 2020). It manifests as a sense of purpose and the ability to invest in professional, intellectual, and recreational interests over time in a dedicated but balanced way.

For Personality Disorder, the sense of purpose can be compromised in various ways. Based on identity issues, the personality disordered individual may experience a "lack of a common thread" in life and, thus, lack of direction and a purpose-driven life. The patient may act without goals and direction, which can manifest itself as changing educational choices and jobs, even after adolescence. They are typically unaware of what they want to achieve or accomplish in life, and this pattern can also contribute to maintaining an existing identity confusion and a deflated sense of self-worth.

> ### Examples of problems with self-direction in internalising versus externalising problems
>
> Individuals with *internalising* problems (e.g., Negative Affectivity and Detachment) will typically show reluctance to pursue goals due to risk aversion, lack of control, and potentially embarrassing situations (e.g., life can be perceived as socially dangerous and risky). Individuals with *externalising* problems (e.g., Dissociality and Disinhibition) will often have goals based solely on personal gain and/or impulsive and short-term gratification. In some cases, people with high grandiosity may be prone to procrastination and stagnation because, on the one hand, they feel special and superior and, on the other hand, they have an underlying fear and shame associated with possible failure. Similarly, people with psychopathy tend to lack realistic long-term goals, which can be linked to their irresponsible and parasitic lifestyle and pathological lies to cover it up.

They may also be people who, due to anxiousness and feelings of inadequacy, live a stunted life where they do not take any chances and do not apply for their dream education or dream job, despite having the qualifications for it. They may be so afraid that it blocks or paralyses their determination, and they get nowhere in life (Simonsen et al., 2022). They can be said to be goal inhibited.

Conversely, there are also people with anankastic and perfectionistic tendencies who are subject to an extreme self-direction that dictates that they must achieve their goals at all costs and increase their productivity to their own inflated standards (Caligor et al., 2018). This is also seen in people suffering from workaholism, who crave a certain recognition from others through achieving specific goals in their professional life (e.g., making their first million or achieving 200 articles on their publication list). Such a rigid and excessive form of self-direction can reflect a rigid and fixed identity. For example, it can characterise a person who, even after the age of 60 years, clings to the idea of one day becoming a famous actor despite numerous indications that the dream will likely never come true. It can also apply to someone with self-aggrandising and grandiose beliefs who only applies for executive positions despite being a recent graduate and having only received rejections on previous applications. See examples of different levels of severity in Table 3.4.

Table 3.4   Examples of severity levels for impaired self-direction

Mild	Ability to set appropriate goals and work towards them is compromised, and there are problems coping with even minor adversity
Moderate	Can easily give up in the face of adversity due to poor emotion regulation Alternatively, can unreasonably pursue goals that have no chance of success
Severe	Is largely unable to set and pursue realistic goals

Interpersonal Aspects

This section defines and exemplifies the four capacities that relate to interpersonal functioning, which include interest in engaging in relationships with others, ability to understand and appreciate others' perspectives (i.e., social cognition and mentalisation), ability to develop and maintain close and mutually satisfying relationships, and ability to manage conflict in relationships. It is important to emphasise that these capacities are naturally intertwined and interpenetrating (e.g., perspective-taking is linked to reciprocity) and interact with aspects of the self (e.g., a negative perception of how others view you is often associated with a self-experience marked by a sense of inferiority). Examples of functional and dysfunctional aspects of interpersonal functioning are shown in Table 3.5.

Table 3.5 Examples of adaptive and maladaptive aspects of interpersonal functioning

Adaptive functioning	Maladaptive functioning
Interest in engaging in relationships with others	Being detached and avoidant Seeking support/confirmation from others Seeking the attention of others
Ability to understand and value the perspectives of others	Ignores or neglects the perspective of others Overthinking what others think and feel
Ability to develop and maintain close and mutually satisfying relationships	Unstable relationships Dominant or submissive
Ability to manage conflict in relationships	Overreacting or avoiding conflict

Interest in Relationships

For everyone, or at least the vast majority of people, an appropriate balance between being alone and being with others is important. With a normal interest in engaging in relationships, there will always be someone to "have your back," which is a natural defense against threats, and it helps prevent loneliness and the vulnerability of being alone (e.g., in the case of physical illness). Of course, how people fulfil this interest in relationships can vary. Some prefer a narrow network of one or two confidential friends, while others need a large and ever-changing social network. Such differences are a reflection of temperamental style more than personality functioning.

In the case of a Personality Disorder, the interest in engaging in relationships can be compromised in different ways, which may be expressed as social avoidance as well as social intrusiveness (Wilson et al., 2017). A starting point may be that the person is distanced, disconnected, or avoidant towards other people. In rare cases, such distance may be due to a lack of interest in, and indifference towards, other people. Other people are simply seen as a disruptive element that creates hassle and noise and are therefore avoided as much as possible. For a large proportion of our patients, their interest in engaging in relationships will be compromised due to concerns about being shamed, criticised, or abused when interacting with others, so they avoid relationships even though they essentially may long for closeness and recognition.

In addition, there are patients for whom interest is compromised by being overly invested in relationships. These can be dependent and overly reliant individuals who do not see themselves as able to stand up for themselves and consistently seek the support of others to make everyday decisions. It can also apply to people who cannot tolerate when they are not being the centre of attention, which often includes an unnaturally intense interest in engaging in encounters and communities. And, finally, there can be a desperate interest in engaging in relationships, often intimate ones, fuelled by a fear of abandonment.

If a clinician wants to uncover the patient's interest in engaging in relationships, a good method is to draw a circle asking the person to place friends and acquaintances at a distance from the centre (representing themselves). Placements of others based on trust and closeness will often show clear patterns such as excessive dependence (too close to the centre), independence (too far away), or a balance in between.

Examples of interest in relationships for Introversion versus Extroversion

Individuals with an *introverted* and reticent nature (e.g., high Detachment and low Disinhibition) may be avoidant and overly shy due to concerns about others' critical observations. Individuals with an *extroverted* and outgoing nature (e.g., low Detachment and high Dissociality) may crave contact for the attention of others. It can be particularly important to consider the range of problems: Do they occur in isolation in certain contexts, such as immediate relationships, or across relationships, such as friends, family, work, leisure and community? When severity is high, most contexts will usually be affected.

Perspective-Taking

The ability to understand and appreciate the perspectives of others is a neutral description of what takes place in social cognition and mentalisation, that is, the ability to imagine what others are thinking and feeling without reading too much between the lines. In general, this capacity is about the ability to infer and reflect on the mental states of others and use this information in personal and social interactions. "Imagining" what others are thinking or feeling is often referred to as the ability to "mentalise" or to have a theory of mind about what is going on in other people's minds (Bateman & Fonagy, 2016). The process occurs primarily outside conscious awareness and is aimed at interpreting and understanding other people's behaviour in terms of mental states (e.g., needs, feelings, desires, beliefs, goals, intentions, and motivations) and making correct inferences about these mental states.

> **Examples of social cognition and mentalisation in internalising versus externalising problems**
>
> Individuals with *internalising* problems (e.g., Negative Affectivity and Detachment) will typically be overly preoccupied with, and hypersensitive to, cues from others that may indicate rejection or criticism. Individuals with *externalising* problems (e.g., Dissociality and Disinhibition) often show a lack of concern for the needs, feelings, and suffering of others and a lack of remorse.

Essentially, this capacity can be compromised in at least two very different ways (Luyten et al., 2020). On the one hand, the person may overlook or struggle to see other people's perspectives, which is known as hypo-mentalisation. On the other hand, the person may read too much into what others are thinking and feeling, often referred to as hyper-mentalization. In other cases, the capacity for mentalisation may be intact but extremely unbalanced; for example, the person may be able to understand the perspective of others but not appreciate it, as is often the case with people characterised by Dissociality. In this case, we can talk about cold mentalisation, where the person has cognitive and instrumental, but not emotional, empathy. Conversely, many personality disordered individuals with social cognition issues exhibit excessive affect in relation to situations and other people. This may be related to repeated experiences of attachment relationships where the person has had to be overly alert in order to adapt to the caregiver's behaviour (McLaren et al., 2022). Table 3.6 shows examples of severity levels of impaired social cognition and mentalisation.

Table 3.6   Examples of severity levels of impaired social cognition and mentalisation

Mild	Limitations in the ability to understand and appreciate the perspective of others (including excessive empathy) create problems in developing close and mutually satisfying relationships
Moderate	Severe limitations in the ability to understand and appreciate the perspective of others hinder the development of close and mutually satisfying relationships
Severe	In addition to severe limitations in mentalising ability, there can be major problems with recognising and acknowledging unwanted emotions (e.g., anger or sadness)

Intimacy and Mutuality

The ability and interest in developing and maintaining close and mutually satisfying relationships is an important evolutionary premise of humanity. Without this capacity, humans would not bond, reproduce themselves, and receive the support and guidance of others (Baumeister & Leary, 1995). It can be directed towards both intimate or romantic relationships as well as close relationships more generally (e.g., to family or a close friend), and towards relationships one both receives from and contributes to ("give-and-take relationships").

Examples of intimacy and reciprocity in internalising versus externalising problems

Individuals with *internalising* issues (e.g., Negative Affectivity and Detachment) will typically be reluctant to engage in relationships with other people unless they are sure of being accepted. In intimate relationships, they may be inhibited with compromised reciprocity and openness due to fear of being ridiculed or shamed. In relationships, they will often end up feeling that they are constantly taking care of others' needs over their own due to an inability to express needs and set boundaries.

Individuals with *externalising* problems (e.g., Dissociality and Disinhibition) will typically not show a genuine interest in the experiences of others, and/or their relationships may be superficial and only serve their own needs. In intimate relationships, they will often be exploitative and deceitful. In other relationships, intimidation and/or domination will be prominent, and they will only cooperate for personal gain without truly considering relationships as reciprocal.

There are basically four types of disorder associated with this capacity (e.g., Bornstein et al., 2010; Navarro-Gómez et al., 2017). First, there may be a reduced ability or courage to develop and maintain close relationships. It could be someone who is inhibited by anxiousness, insecurity, and shame. But it could also be someone who does not feel a natural desire to get to know other people or to let someone else get to know their real thoughts and feelings. They may have a hard time opening up to another person and consequently have a compromised ability to get close to a spouse, friend, or partner. Often the person will also feel lonely even when in the company of others.

Second, there may be intense, unstable, and turbulent intimate relationships. This pattern will often be closely linked to dysfunction in the other capacities. In such cases, the person may feel overly attached to a partner in an unhealthy and dependent way. This can leave them feeling lost and desperate when alone or constantly seeking a relationship to feel admired. Quite often, people with moderate to severe levels of personality dysfunction can feel so fearful of rejection or abandonment that they push their partner away or break up to avoid the pain or engage in a kick-and-cling dynamic. In the most severe cases, individuals only interact or bond with other people when absolutely necessary. Finally, this capacity will often also manifest in the individual's sexuality, particularly in the ability to integrate sexuality with emotional intimacy (e.g., combining tenderness or play with eroticism).

Third, it can involve intimate relationships where the person with a Personality Disorder assumes the submissive and self-effacing role, which in the most serious cases can include violence and abuse, without the person being able to speak up or keep themselves safe. It is a relationship where the person gives without getting anything in return, while the other party simply exploits and receives.

Finally, there may be the reverse constellation, where the person with a Personality Disorder dominates, exploits, and takes advantage of the close relationships they are involved in. This may be an opportunistic or parasitic behaviour that the person generally uses in their relationships with others; for example, instead of providing means for the household, the person relies on a hard-working partner, where they always find shelter and food on the table. Table 3.7 shows examples of severity levels of disrupted intimacy and reciprocity.

Table 3.7   Examples of severity levels of disrupted intimacy and reciprocity

Mild	Relationships can be characterised by a lack of reciprocity, for example in the form of dependency, where the person is indulgent to a degree that comes at a significant cost to themselves.
Moderate	Persistent problems in all relationships, which can be very one-sided, for example, the person is very dominant or very submissive.
Severe	To the extent the person has relationships, these lack reciprocity and are superficial, extremely one-sided and unstable Family relationships are typically absent (despite living relatives).

Conflict Management

As a natural extension of being able to establish and maintain mutually satisfying relationships, it is also essential to be able to handle conflicts in these relationships in a healthy way, neither accepting too much nor too little. In practice, it is all about the art of choosing your battles wisely, which is also referred to as assertiveness in terms of not being overly submissive or too aggressive (e.g., Speed et al., 2018). Sometimes it is better to stand firm in an argument even though it causes tension, while other times the opposite is true. Conflict management is, of course, vital to maintaining stable cooperative relationships, whether this pertains to family or work life. People with significant problems with this can find it difficult to socialise with others. Some people may struggle because they are stubborn and basically do not want to listen to other people's opinions. Others may struggle with conflict management due to affect lability and problems with mentalisation, and there may also be some who stifle their own needs and opinions out of an excessive longing for togetherness and stability.

In more severe cases of disorder, there may be a one-sided approach to conflict management, where the person always gives up in a conflict-avoidant manner, while the partner gets their way. This can be an exhausting and self-defeating pattern that goes hand in hand with a lack of reciprocity. Conversely, there can also be a different kind of one-sided conflict management, where the person with a Personality Disorder is the one who must consistently be right in every discussion in order to keep the peace, which means that everyone around them must submit and "walk on eggshells" in order not to cause a fuss. Individuals with such tendencies may refrain from cooperating with others altogether due to widespread distrust or a complete lack of altruism.

> **Examples of conflict management in internalising versus externalising problems**
>
> People with *internalising* problems (e.g., Negative Affectivity and Detachment) may tend to avoid conflict in order to "please" others, at the expense of their own needs. People with *externalising* problems (e.g., Dissociality and Disinhibition) may be inclined to seek out or provoke conflict, either because they get a "kick" out of it and/or because it gives them a sense of power.

To summarise, there are those who overreact and perhaps get a "kick" out of a good conflict, while others underreact and avoid conflict, which is especially harmful in the long run. In some cases, the same person can be submissive in one relationship and overreact and dominate in another. People with healthy personality functioning will often strive for balanced conflict management, that is, show a certain flexibility in being able to stand their ground, but also be able to back down and recognise their own faults and shortcomings. When a clinician is interested in uncovering this capacity, it will be natural to ask about specific conflict situations and thus get a picture of the person's inclinations both in the situation itself and in resolving the conflict. Table 3.8 shows examples of severity levels of disturbed conflict management ability.

Table 3.8   Examples of severity levels of disrupted conflict management skills

Mild	Relationships are usually characterised by periodic or frequent minor conflicts that are not so severe that they lead to serious or long-term break-ups. Alternatively, relationships can be characterised by conflict avoidance, where the person is compliant to a degree that comes at some cost to themselves.
Moderate	Tendency to more frequent, severe, and explosive conflicts.
Severe	To the extent that the person has relationships, they are highly conflicted, often to the point of violence and self-harm. Family relationships are absent, if not marred by significant conflict.

Emotional Manifestations

As already described, the severity of Personality Disorder is determined not only by compromised personality functioning (e.g., inferiority and poor understanding of others' perspectives), but also by how the dysfunction manifests itself both emotionally (e.g., emotional overreaction to small setbacks), cognitively (e.g., unrealistic or psychotic interpretations in stressful situations), and behaviourally (e.g., self-harm as an attempt to regulate difficult emotions). Specifically, it is the severity and rigidity of these manifestations that must be considered when assessing severity. Most people can sometimes exhibit some of these manifestations (e.g., emotional overreaction or paralysis in a specific but relatively rare situation) without this necessarily constituting a consistent emotional pattern.

It is important to consider the manifestations as naturally intertwined and connected to the basic capacities as well as to individual trait dispositions. For example, it is very natural that people with predominant Negative Affectivity (e.g., emotional lability) have a deficient ability to maintain an overall positive self-esteem and often exhibit emotional manifestations in the form of being emotionally overreactive and uncertain about decision making. In the next three sections, we will first outline the emotional manifestations of personality functioning, which include emotional range and appropriateness, under- and over-regulation of emotions, and the ability to recognise one's own emotions.

Emotional Range and Appropriateness

Feelings usually refer to the conscious experience of emotions, while the latter is often understood more broadly to include both pre-conscious and more biologically based responses. Emotions add colour and meaning to life, but they can also become overwhelming and lead to poor decisions and inappropriate behaviour. Emotion regulation enables humans to both experience a full range of emotions (e.g., sadness, anger, fear, joy, and contempt) while keeping our emotions under control in a given situation and in accordance with cultural and contextual expectations and norms. Disruptions in emotional range and appropriateness can manifest as both a lack of capacity to experience specific feelings or to integrate multiple relevant feelings, simultaneously (e.g., Carpenter & Trull, 2013; Lynch et al., 2015; Solbakken et al., 2011). This will often result in emotional responses not being expressed in a healthy and appropriate way (e.g., not feeling appropriately angry or not integrating tender feelings with anger when appropriately upset by close others).

Under- and Over-Regulation of Emotions

Emotion regulation is a crucial capacity in humans, as emotions are known to be a vital driver of our well-being, relationships, and survival. People with emotional dysregulation often feel hypersensitive to situations or people, both positively and negatively. When the ability to regulate emotions is intact, the person may use mature coping strategies, including self-regulation, intentional suppression, or sublimation of difficult emotions, whereas impaired emotion regulation may be associated with more immature defense mechanisms such as repression, displacement, dissociation, and projection (Caligor et al., 2018; Linehan, 1993).

Essentially, Personality Disorder is characterised by at least two types of compromised emotion regulation (e.g., Blay et al., 2024; D'Aurizio et al., 2023; Frederiksen et al., 2021). On the one hand, individuals with Personality Disorder may find that they cannot control their emotions, which causes them serious problems with other people (e.g., explosiveness). On the other hand, some people with Personality Disorders may also be emotionally withdrawn, closed off, or over-controlled to the extent that others complain about their lack of emotional expression (e.g., Lynch et al., 2015). In complex and more severe cases, the same person may oscillate between under- and over-regulation; for example, alternating between dissociative and projective defenses.

Recognising Own Emotions

This capacity relates to the ability to not only recognise but also acknowledge difficult or unwanted emotions (e.g., anger and sadness). The aforementioned capacity for emotion regulation is supported by the individual's ability to recognise, acknowledge, symbolise, or mentalise affectively meaningful experiences (i.e., represent the emotion mentally rather than behaviourally) and to "think before acting" (Bateman & Fonagy, 2016). The ability to recognise one's own emotions therefore also involves being able to integrate and verbalise affect states correctly, including the unwanted or unpleasant ones.

A specific term often used to describe deficiencies in ability to recognise one's own emotions is alexithymia (Taylor & Bagby, 2012). Many people with Personality Disorder have alexithymia, meaning they lack words or are blind to their own emotions. Alexithymia is in itself a dimensional phenomenon and not an either/or concept. People vary and are more or less good at differentiating between different emotional states and generally have varying degrees of interest in emotional life. Alexithymia can be divided into three components, which will often interact with each other. First, it is an inability to identify emotions, that is, to consciously feel the emotions (e.g., physically). Second, someone may be able to identify emotions but have great difficulty describing them; for example, all emotions are simply referred to with generic words such as annoying, frustrating, or stressful. Third, there may be a tendency to be externalising, which in this context means that the person shows little attention and interest in their emotional life and tends to focus on the physical and concrete instead. Much psychotherapeutic treatment is aimed at increasing a person's ability to feel and verbalise their emotions, and this can in many cases be an essential component for improving personality functioning (Simonsen et al., 2021).

In some cases, difficulties in recognising one's own unwanted emotions (e.g., anger over the way the boss has treated you) can be expressed by displacing the emotion on to a more secure person (e.g., spouse or close friend) who then becomes the object of the anger instead. In a more severe Personality Disorder, one's own unwanted emotions (e.g., anger or jealousy) can be attributed to other people in the form of projective identification (Caligor et al., 2018). For example, in a stressful situation, the person may perceive or interpret that others are angry with them, when in fact they themselves are experiencing unwanted feelings of anger. In practice, the recipient of the projection can be subtly pressured or manipulated to behave in accordance with the projected theme (e.g., anger), which in itself maintains interpersonal dysfunction.

Cognitive Manifestations

As mentioned, the severity of a Personality Disorder is determined not only by how the dysfunction manifests itself emotionally but also cognitively (e.g., unrealistic or psychotic perceptions in stressful situations). In the next three sections, we will therefore outline the cognitive manifestations of personality functioning, which include reality testing, decision making and judgement, as well as stability and flexibility of beliefs.

Reality Testing

The description "accuracy of situational and interpersonal appraisals, especially under stress" is a neutral definition of what is traditionally called "reality testing" (Hurvich, 1970). The ability to distinguish our inner world from reality is something that we use more or less constantly in our everyday life. Imagine you just said hello to a colleague at work, but they did not respond and looked a bit grumpy. Your first thought might be that your colleague was angry with you for some reason. But because your capacity for "reality testing" is intact, you quickly realise that your colleague may not have seen you, was lost in thought, had a stomach ache, or was grumpy because of personal concerns. In line with this example, you can also imagine one of your patients who is desperate because her boyfriend has not texted her for almost 3 hours and also is not responding to her calls. Your patient might conclude that her boyfriend must have left her and found someone else who he suddenly met. But, in reality, your patient has not received a message or call from her boyfriend because his mobile phone has run out of battery.

So far, these examples reflect a kind of breakdown in mentalising ability or interpersonal appraisals. But if we imagine an even higher level of impaired reality testing, we may face something akin to delusions and psychosis, because it is on the verge of a fully fledged psychotic state, where perception takes on a more absolute character (D'Agostino et al., 2019).

Reality testing traditionally refers to people's ability to distinguish their inner thoughts, feelings, and ideas from real-life events. Successful reality testing involves seeing a situation as it really is, rather than what you hope or fear it might be. We can all locate our perceptions on such a spectrum, ranging from a shared reality to a private reality. The concept of reality testing is an important marker for different levels of personality pathology (Caligor et al., 2018).

In the most severe Personality Disorders, it is quite common to see transient loss of reality testing, either in highly stressful or emotionally charged situations, or if the individual is under the influence of drugs and/or alcohol. It should be noted that persistent loss of reality testing is not characteristic of Personality Disorder but should lead to further investigation for a Psychotic Disorder. Diagnosis of Personality Disorder should generally not be made when a person is characterised by an acute condition. However, in individuals with severe personality dysfunction, transient psychotic-like experiences may be normal due to a highly vulnerable and disintegrated internal personality structure combined with highly immature coping strategies (Caligor et al., 2018). These typically occur in the context of high affect, stress, dissociation, and reminders of childhood trauma, where symptoms are not only activated but can also intensify (Beatson et al., 2019; D'Agostino et al., 2019; Tseng & Georgiades, 2024). In contrast, schizophreniform symptoms such as formal thought disorders, bizarre delusions, and negative symptoms are unlikely to be related to severity of personality dysfunction. The same is usually also true for somatic and grandiose delusions and other persistent hallucinations (Beatson et al., 2019).

As a psychopathological process, compromised reality testing can have a very concrete experiential quality that occurs when the person experiences some form of emotional pressure. In such cases, their immediate experience (e.g., suspicion and perceived threat) is all there is. It is in this moment that the experience takes on the quality of absolute reality. In this situation, from the patient's perspective, there is no distinction between their own internal and external reality. What they think and feel is simply judged and experienced as absolute reality, leaving no room for alternative perspectives. Such a manifestation of weakened reality testing is essentially similar to Harry S. Sullivan's (1968) concept of "parataxic distortion," in which misperceptions of others can be based on past experiences and projected fantasies. According to Kernberg's theory of how personality organises itself at different levels of disturbance, reality testing is defined as the ability to evaluate conventional notions of reality (Caligor et al., 2018). When individuals with Severe Personality Disorder experience emotional pressure, they may be drawn into a "private reality" from time to time. In mentalisation theory, this state is described as the result of the primary unconscious, resulting in a disruption of consciousness and normal intentionality and motivation (Fonagy & Allison, 2016).

A Mild Personality Disorder may involve what cognitive behavioural therapy refers to as cognitive distortions, where individuals who are under stress and pressure may expect the worst to happen (i.e., catastrophic thinking) or easily feel rejected by criticism from others (Freeman & Beck, 1990). In this way, mildly impaired reality testing is not fundamentally different from the cognitive distortions associated with depression and anxiety. In a Severe Personality Disorder, the magnitude of these distortions is significantly increased, so that under pressure the person can lose touch with reality; for example, in the form of extreme paranoid perceptions, out-of-body experiences, or seeing or hearing something that others do not. In addition to differences in experiential quality, the degree of reality testing must also be seen in the context of the personality's other capacities that can have a reinforcing or modifying influence. See Table 3.9 for examples of severity levels of disordered reality testing.

Assessment of reality testing may be one of the components in personality assessment where clinicians need to have relatives involved in the assessment process, because in many cases it can be both difficult and shameful for the person to remember. In addition, the clinician must pay particular attention to asking about episodes where the person has been exposed to severe distress. An important focus here will be to highlight differences and similarities in how the person perceives the situation here and now compared to then and there.

Table 3.9   Examples of severity levels of disrupted reality testing under stress

Mild	There may be some distortion in the person's situational and interpersonal appraisals, but reality testing typically remains essentially intact.
Moderate	There may be considerable distortion in the person's situational and interpersonal appraisals as well as the presence of mild dissociative states or psychotic-like beliefs or perceptions (e.g., paranoid ideas).
Severe	There may be extreme distortions in the person's situational and interpersonal appraisal as well as frequently occurring dissociative states or psychotic-like beliefs or perceptions (e.g., extremely paranoid reactions).

Decision Making in Uncertain Situations

As a natural manifestation of healthy personality functioning, including stability of identity, a well-regulated emotional life, a realistic assessment of one's strengths and weaknesses, an overall stable and positive self-esteem, and a flexible capacity for self-direction, there will also be a healthy ability to make appropriate decisions in situations of uncertainty.

As pointed out by the Canadian philosopher Charles Taylor (1989), our sense of identity enables us to judge what is important for us and what is not. Such a "meaning making system" provides us with a framework for decision making according to what is good, true, and valuable, which eventually helps us stick to our decisions, and reach our goals, even in very uncertain situations (Taylor, 1989). Individuals with a poorly integrated sense of identity, including overall stable beliefs and values, therefore tend to experience everything as equally important resulting in paralysis, confusion, and inconsistency in their decision making. This is often painful and complicates relationships with other people (McAdams, 2020).

Decision making can also be considered a central component in self-regulatory and self-directing efforts where fear of shame, not measuring up, and falling short may typically lead to decision-making problems (Ronningstam & Baskin-Sommers, 2013). Thus, disordered personality functioning often involves an inadequate ability to make appropriate decisions in uncertain situations, which can manifest as a lack of integrity, autonomy, and agency when under pressure (McAdams, 2020). Decision making and judgement are particularly closely linked to a person's identity and sense of purpose in that decisions and judgement are situated and thus linked to the sense of connection between present and future. The person orientates towards the future (e.g., achieving a goal or resolving a conflict) by adapting to the present (e.g., choosing peace over justice). This manifestation is an expression of the strategies that are adapted and utilised in the here and now to achieve a more important long-term goal (e.g., peace and amity).

Difficulties with decision making and judgement are typically seen in interpersonally dependent individuals, who have particular difficulty making decisions without seeking advice and support from others, including everyday situations such as what food to order at a restaurant. In practice, some people with these difficulties can become so ambivalent or paralysed that they are unable to make a decision or they choose to procrastinate. Perhaps such paralysis can feel unsafe in itself? Perhaps shame will emerge as a reaction to not making a decision about something that is entirely one's own responsibility? Decision-making issues may often be seen in those with narcissistic personality dysfunction because of their hypersensitivity to fear, shame, and failure (Ronningstam & Baskin-Sommers, 2013). Finally, some individuals with Personality Disorder may end up making inappropriate or ill-considered decisions based on poor judgement in situations of uncertainty (e.g., moving in with a charming person they just met) or in other ways being reckless in their decision making. This is somewhat supported by research showing that individuals with pronounced Personality Disorder tend to make more disadvantaged decisions in experimental tests and have difficulty resisting an impulse to take an immediately available reward in the hope of obtaining a better reward in the future (Paret et al., 2017).

Stability and Flexibility of Beliefs

As previously described in relation to identity, healthy personality functioning will usually be characterised by a coherent and stable sense of identity, which involves a consistent sense of self and a well-integrated interaction between different aspects of the person. Thus, in the case of personality dysfunction, there will either be significant variation, instability, or contradiction in self-view and identity ("missing the common thread"), or identity and self-view may be overly rigid and fixed. As a natural cognitive manifestation of this, healthy personality functioning involves appropriate stability and flexibility in beliefs, while disordered personality functioning may involve overly fluid and inconsistent beliefs with an absence of personal integrity ("chameleon effect") or overly rigid or unwavering beliefs about oneself and/or other people. A person with a strong identity confusion and lack of independence may tend to adopt the beliefs, preferences, and opinions of others in terms of clothing style, musical tastes, or political orientation, which often results in the person not having their own point of view on life. Conversely, you may also meet patients who are stuck in a belief that has not really helped them move forward in life in a healthy way; for example, a 62-year-old man who has had a lifelong belief that he is a talented actor who just needs to be discovered by the film industry. Such a person is highly inflexible and thus has a vulnerable foundation in life that can easily crumble beneath them if their illusions are shattered one day. This essential perspective sheds light on the personality's "ideological framework" (McAdams, 2020), which constitutes fundamental values and beliefs that, when disrupted, can lead to recurrent identity crises.

Behavioural Manifestations

The severity of a Personality Disorder is determined not only by how the dysfunction manifests itself emotionally and cognitively, but also behaviourally (e.g., self-harm as an attempt to regulate difficult emotions). In the next two sections, we will therefore outline the behavioural manifestations of personality dysfunction, which include impulse and behavioural control, and behavioural responses including harm to self and others.

Impulse and Behavioural Control

Flexibility in impulse control and adapting behaviour to the situation while taking potential consequences into account are important for a functional life. A well-functioning person can act spontaneously when necessary while maintaining appropriate control over their own impulses and actions. From an evolutionary perspective, it would never have worked if everyone in the tribe had been restrained and inhibited when there was a sudden opportunity to take down a prey animal that could ensure the tribe's survival. At the same time, it would never have worked if everyone in the tribe had spontaneously scurried around at the slightest impulse or distraction. The ideal balance may include a little bit of both, depending on the situation, and it can be an advantage that some people are more inclined to one thing and others to another. All things being equal, it can be assumed that an individual with courage, risk-taking behaviour, and potent actions have endowed the tribe with advantages and the individual with a certain recognition, power, and position.

In the case of Personality Disorder such advantages seem less evident. On the one hand, you will see people who often act so rashly or impulsively that it causes them serious problems or even severe and lethal harm (Sebastian et al., 2013). They may take risks that endanger themselves or others both physically, financially, and psychologically (e.g., gambling, promiscuity, risky behaviour in traffic). On the other hand, you can see people who tend to be so over-controlled in their actions that they fail to recognise the many spontaneous opportunities that arise in life (Lynch et al., 2015). Their restrictions and inhibitions stifle their ability to have a fulfilling life.

Behavioural Reactions Including Harm to Self and Others

In healthy personality functioning, there will usually be appropriate behavioural responses to intense emotions and stressful circumstances. As a manifestation of disordered personality functioning, problems with such reactions are typically seen in the form of self-harm and interpersonal aggression. This is associated with emotion dysregulation or, more specifically, underregulation of intense and difficult emotions. Instead of feeling or enduring such difficult emotions, the patient may automatically resort to "acting out," where internal emotional tension is not remembered, experienced, or verbalised, but is expressed as violent or impulsive actions. Finally, interpersonal aggression can also act as a "defense" against other people who are getting too close, which activates or reveals the patient's underlying vulnerability (Horney, 2013). Simply put, some patients may find that aggression serves as their best defense. See Table 3.10 for examples of severity levels of harm to oneself or other people.

Table 3.10 Examples of severity levels of harm to self or others

Mild	Typically not associated with significant harm to self or others
Moderate	Sometimes associated with harm to self or others
Severe	Often associated with harm to self or others

In most clinical settings, it has become routine to encounter patients who self-harm in one way or another. As a common denominator, the majority of the aforementioned capacities and manifestations are in play. There will typically be a pattern of impaired emotion regulation, increased emotional reactivity, impaired mentalisation, lack of recognition of own emotions (alexithymia), poor impulse control, negative self-perception, and a high level of perfectionism, inferiority, and shame (Rubæk & Møhl, 2023). Typically, all aspects of personality functioning will be disturbed when self-harm is present. Table 3.11 shows a number of aspects of how self-harm can be expressed and the function it may serve (Rubæk & Møhl, 2023). On the one hand, self-harm can include victimisation, such as allowing oneself to be sexually exploited or abused. On the other hand, it may involve the patient directly causing harm to themselves using sharp objects or the like.

Table 3.11 Examples of different aspects of self-harm

Suicidal self-harm Done with the intention to die	What is the intention? <---------------------->	**Non-suicidal** No desire to die, hope for psychological recovery
Indirect harm Often over time	How immediate? <---------------------->	**Direct harm** Often immediate
Self-harm by proxy The person intentionally causes another person to harm themselves	Who inflicts it? <---------------------->	**Self-inflicted self-harm** The person themselves
Self-harm with cultural acceptance For example, extensive tattooing, piercing, and extreme sports	How socially acceptable? <---------------------->	**Self-harm without cultural acceptance** For example, excessive alcohol consumption or banging your head against the wall
Digital self-harm Destructive online behaviour with psychological harm	Physical or virtual? <---------------------->	**Physical self-harm** Destructive offline behaviour with physical harm

Psychosocial Impairment and Distress

In addition to aspects of self and interpersonal dysfunction, as well as emotional, cognitive, and behavioural manifestations, it is also necessary to assess the global psychosocial level of functioning and level of distress before determining whether a Personality Disorder is actually present and how severe it is. Specifically, the focus is on the extent to which dysfunction in the aforementioned areas is associated with suffering or impairment in personal, family, social, educational, occupational, or other significant areas of functioning. This reflects the World Health Organization's fundamental focus on psychosocial impairment and distress as crucial factors in making a mental health diagnosis (Reed, 2024). Otherwise, it would easily lead to overdiagnosis and pathologisation of otherwise normal conditions and reactions (Paris, 2015). In the next three sections, we will therefore seek to clarify how psychosocial functioning and distress should be understood in relation to the diagnosis of Personality Disorder. An overview of how this can be expressed at different levels of severity is shown in Table 3.12.

Table 3.12 Overview of psychosocial functioning for different severity levels of Personality Disorder

Personality Difficulty	Typically associated with certain problems with functioning in life, but these are not of sufficient severity to cause noticeable disruption in social, occupational, and interpersonal relationships, or they are limited to specific relationships or situations.
Mild Personality Disorder	May be associated with distress or impairment in personal, family, social, educational, occupational, or other significant areas of functioning that are either limited to specific areas (e.g., relationships or work) or is present in multiple areas to a lesser degree.
Moderate Personality Disorder	Associated with significant impairment in personal, family, social, educational, occupational, or other significant areas of functioning, although some level of functioning in limited areas may be preserved.
Severe Personality Disorder	Associated with severe impairment in all or almost all areas of life, including personal, family, social, educational, employment, or other significant areas of functioning.

Dysfunction and Distress Must Be Attributed to Personality Disturbances

A non-disordered personality is characterised by sufficient flexibility to respond appropriately and adapt to other people's behaviour, life events, and changes in the environment, which therefore does not involve psychosocial impairment or significant distress in itself. However, if psychosocial impairment and distress do occur in such cases, it should not be interpreted as a sign of an underlying Personality Disorder, but most likely a distressing psychological condition (e.g., Adjustment Disorder, Post Traumatic Stress Disorder, or depression) or physical condition (e.g., Parkinson's disease or chronic pain). When psychosocial impairment or distress is attributable to Personality Disorder, it is because aspects of the self and interpersonal dysfunction and cognitive, emotional, and behavioural patterns themselves are so maladaptive (e.g., inflexible or poorly regulated) that they cause significant distress or impairment in personal, family, social, educational, occupational, and other important aspects of functioning. The clinician needs to make this connection explicit when diagnosing Personality Disorder. This is achieved by specific questions such as "Did this difficulty with not having a clear sense of who you are make you distressed or upset?" or "In which situations did this problem with handling emotions cause you problems?" The clinician uses their clinical judgement to determine whether or not the answers provided to such questions are sufficient for meeting the requirements for dysfunction and/or distress. This can sometimes be challenging as we might have different norms for what characterises a well-functioning person (Kiel, Lind et al., 2024).

Temporary or Situationally Impaired Psychosocial Functioning

In terms of psychosocial functioning, ICD-11 emphasises that personality disturbances *should* manifest across a range of personal and social situations over an extended period of time (e.g., 2 or more years) to warrant a diagnosis of Personality Disorder. Behavioural patterns that only appear in the context of specific relationships, social roles, settings, or circumstances, or patterns that have only lasted for a short period of time, are therefore not a sufficient basis for diagnosing a Personality Disorder. Instead, the likelihood that such behaviours are a response to psychosocial circumstances (e.g., divorce, life crisis, being fired from one's job) must be considered. In such cases, focus on problems in the relevant relationships or circumstances (e.g., family or school) may be more appropriate than the diagnosis of Personality Disorder.

When Psychosocial Dysfunction and Distress Affects Others

With the aforementioned clarified, it is relevant to take a closer look at the meaning of psychosocial impairment because, in addition to the people who experience psychosocial disability and distress themselves, it can also be something that greatly affects relatives or colleagues. In Personality Disorder, examples show that people with predominant trait features of Dissociality can be fearless, self-promoting, reckless, and seemingly successful at the expense of other people's safety and well-being. Personality disordered individuals with prominent Dissociality often do not express a lot of distress or negative emotions, which can be attributed to the stress immunity that often characterises their pattern of Personality Disorder. On the one hand, such individuals may hold high-ranking titles (e.g., president or chief executive officer), which would seem to reflect a high level of psychosocial functioning. On the other hand, they can destroy and poison their environment with manipulation, threats, and psychological, physical, or sexual intimidation. In such cases, it is the people around the personality disordered individual who experience both distress and psychosocial impairment. To some extent, the same can also apply to people with predominant Anankastia, where resources, discipline, self-control, overview, and strong goal orientation are often present. Such people tend to do well in education and employment, while relatives or colleagues may "suffer" from the person's way of functioning and acting. Ultimately, this can evidently lead to conflicts and, in turn, psychosocial problems for the individual too.

Chapter 4
Severity Classification

The assessment of aspects of self and interpersonal dysfunction as well as emotional, cognitive, and behavioural manifestations (see Chapter 3) can result in five different levels of severity or personality functioning, and it is also possible to diagnose a Personality Disorder without specifying the severity.

0. No personality disturbance
1. Personality Difficulty (subthreshold)
2. Personality Disorder, mild
3. Personality Disorder, moderate
4. Personality Disorder, severe
Z. Personality Disorder, severity unspecified

In this chapter, the different levels of personality dysfunction in ICD-11 are provided. In addition, we have added illustrative cases for each level of severity. For clarity, we refer to Table 4.1, which presents an abbreviated overview of what characterises the different levels of severity.

Table 4.1   Abbreviated overview of characteristics of Personality Disorder severity levels

Mild	Moderate	Severe
Affects only *some aspects* of the self (e.g., self-esteem) or all functions but to a lesser degree.	Affects *multiple* aspects of self-functioning (e.g., self-esteem, identity, and purposefulness).	Severe impact on *virtually all* aspects of self-functioning. For example, self-view may be highly unstable or governed by self-loathing, extreme rigidity, or self-overestimation.
Problems in *many* interpersonal relationships, while some relationships and roles are preserved.	Significant problems in *most* interpersonal relationships and roles.	Severe problems in *virtually all* relationships where the ability or willingness to fulfil social or work roles is severely compromised or absent.

Table 4.1 Continued

Mild	Moderate	Severe
Some relationships may be characterised by distance, periodic minor conflicts, dependency and conflict avoidance (e.g., being compliant to a degree that comes at some cost to the person).	Existing relationships can be characterised by frequent, severe, or explosive conflicts or they can be very one-sided (e.g., the person is very dominant or very submissive).	The relationships that do exist lack reciprocity or are superficial, extremely one-sided, unstable, or highly conflictual, often to the point of violence.
Under stress, there may be some distortion in the person's situational and interpersonal judgement (e.g., catastrophising), but reality testing typically remains intact.	Under stress, mild dissociative states or psychotic-like beliefs or perceptions (e.g., paranoid ideas) may occur.	Under stress, dissociative states or psychotic-like beliefs or perceptions can often occur (e.g., extremely paranoid reactions).
Typically, not associated with significant harm to self or others.	Sometimes associated with harm to self or others.	Often associated with harm to self or others.

Personality Difficulty

We begin here with the sub-diagnostic category of Personality Difficulty, which does not describe a diagnosis or mental disorder, but instead appears as a possible code related to problems with interpersonal interaction that may affect the person's health status and contact with the healthcare system. This is in many ways comparable to the non-diagnostic ICD-10 code for "Accentuated personality traits" (Z73.1). Personality Difficulty refers to pronounced personality characteristics that may affect treatment or healthcare, but without reaching a level that gives rise to a diagnosis. Personality Difficulty is characterised by long-standing disturbances (e.g., at least 2 years) in the individual's way of experiencing and thinking about the self, others, and the world. In contrast to a Personality Disorder, the presence of Personality Difficulty is only intermittently manifested in cognitive and emotional experience and expression (e.g., during times of stress) or at low intensity. Personality Difficulty is typically associated with some problems in functioning, but these are insufficiently severe to cause notable disruption in social, occupational, and interpersonal relationships or may be limited to specific relationships or situations. By becoming familiar with this sub-diagnostic category of severity, the clinician also realises that the threshold between diagnosis and non-diagnosis is not a distinction between "disturbed" and "healthy." As we will see in the following case examples, it takes more than just personality difficulties to be diagnosed with a Personality Disorder.

Case: Ellen

Ellen is a slightly introverted 25-year-old single woman who is finishing her first year of nursing school. She previously studied literature at the university but dropped out because she could no longer see herself in the subject matter.

Like many of her high school classmates, Ellen has struggled to figure out what to do with her life. Her friends call her a perfectionist because she is always striving for top grades, and they feel she is more concerned with academic achievement than living a good life.

While most of her friends have graduated from university, Ellen is unfulfilled in terms of her life goals. At university, she did not achieve the same level of academic success as she did in high school, causing her to question her own abilities and ambitions. During the same period, she broke up with her boyfriend after a 2-year relationship. She has kept in touch with two close friends from high school, but often feels jealous that they have found their path in life and are now getting married. However, she never expresses any of these feelings to her friends, but rather tends to get a little annoyed with them and feel somewhat sad inside.

Thus, Ellen mostly keeps her difficult emotions to herself and withdraws from close relationships, while anxiously pushing herself harder professionally. One day she hopes to become an extraordinarily skilled nurse that people will admire.

Case: Tim

Tim is an energetic 41-year-old medical doctor who recently landed his dream position at a prestigious hospital's orthopaedic surgery department. He lives with his stay-at-home wife, with whom he has two young children.

Tim has always liked challenges and competition and, in this context, he can sometimes get a little mischievous, especially if he feels he is being outdone by others. For example, he has successfully completed two marathons, mainly because he wanted to beat one of his colleagues' records.

At work, Tim also tends to compete with colleagues to be the most efficient or have the most correct views on professional issues, which occasionally involves a disrespectful and harsh tone. Quite often, he stays at work late into the night in order to live up to the standards he sets for himself.

On weekends, he often spends time with a group of friends with whom he competes in various challenges. Tim's wife often complains about his fanatical commitment to work and competitive sports at the expense of his family. She feels he rarely considers her perspective on things. In turn, he feels she has unreasonably high expectations and wants to control him.

Mild Personality Disorder

In a Mild Personality Disorder, there are usually only some areas of the self that are impaired, while other areas are preserved. For example, there may be problems with self-direction, but not so much with stability in the sense of identity or self-esteem. At this mild level of severity, all areas may also be impaired to a lesser degree and the disorder may not necessarily be evident in all contexts. Thus, problems may occur in many interpersonal relationships and manifest in the way the person fulfils expected occupational or social roles, but some relationships are maintained and/or some social roles are fulfilled. Mild Personality Disorder is typically not associated with substantial harm to self or others. However, it may be associated with significant distress or with impairment in personal, family, social, educational, or occupational functioning or other important areas of functioning that are either limited to circumscribed areas (e.g., romantic relationships, employment) or present in more areas but of milder severity.

In Mild Personality Disorder, the person's sense of self may be somewhat contradictory or inconsistent with how other people view them. There may be difficulties recovering from experiences that have injured their self-esteem. The person's ability to set appropriate goals and work towards them is compromised and they have difficulty handling even minor setbacks. The person may have conflicts with supervisors and co-workers but is generally able to sustain employment in such cases. Their limited ability to understand and appreciate the perspectives of others creates difficulties in developing close and mutually satisfying relationships. Some relationships may be characterised by estrangement, but relationships are more commonly characterised by intermittent or frequent conflicts that are not so severe that they cause any serious or long-standing disruption. Alternatively, relationships may be characterised by dependence and conflict avoidance by giving in to others, even at some cost to themselves. Under stress, there may be some distortions in the individual's situational and interpersonal appraisals (e.g., catastrophising in slightly stressful situations), but reality testing typically remains intact. The next two case examples are meant to illustrate how a Mild Personality Disorder can manifest itself and are by no means exhaustive.

Case: Elizabeth

Elizabeth is a 43-year-old single woman who is very deliberate and clear about what she wants in life and what she expects from others. After a serious car accident, Elizabeth has developed symptoms of Post Traumatic Stress Disorder and is referred for assessment and treatment in the public healthcare system.

Her counsellor discovers that Elizabeth has ended several relationships. She never feels her partners are good enough for her because they do not live up to her standards and are obstacles on her career path. The men she initially finds charming, she soon realises are rude and repulsive. She has started to think that there are no "good" men out there and that she will always be alone.

Elizabeth has a master's degree in public administration and worked as a consultant in an office where she was considered a good employee by her immediate managers. However, she criticised her colleagues' laziness and could become pedantic when others were not efficient or precise enough in their communication. After complaints from colleagues to the human resource department, a staff dispute was opened against her. Instead of defending herself, Elizabeth quit her job, determined to work as an independent consultant. Her car accident occurred shortly after this decision.

At the first clinical consultation, Elizabeth acts somewhat defensively. She avoids answering questions about her personality, her childhood, or her close relationships, saying she does not see how this could be relevant to her case. She repeatedly criticises the therapist for not being on time and not being eloquent enough. She emphasises her own prestigious academic and employment history, while questioning the therapist's credentials and intellectual ability.

Case: Tobias

Tobias is an introverted 37-year-old graphic designer in a relationship with a slightly older woman with whom he has two children.

Tobias was bullied at school, while his parents failed to protect him due to their own issues with anxiety and alcoholism. At times, his father was explosive and verbally threatening, especially after consuming alcohol. Tobias gradually withdrew both in the home and at school to avoid situations where he could be hurt or humiliated.

He is a nervous and sensitive nature, and he expects others to think negatively about him. Although he was successful as a freelance web and graphic designer for small businesses and was in a long-term relationship, he continues to struggle with emotional issues as an adult and was referred to a psychologist for treatment of recurring episodes of depression and anxiety complicated by self-medicating with cannabis.

This pattern has particularly arisen because his work situation requires regular interaction with colleagues, which significantly increases his anxiousness. In addition, Tobias often works overtime without demanding any payment for it. On the one hand, this alleviates his concerns about whether his efforts are good enough, but it also causes him to feel exploited and stressed.

In his private life, Tobias is often in a submissive role to his partner, doing everything she asks out of concern that she will leave him, even in situations with pressing deadlines at work. The pressures of both work and home life have led Tobias to increasingly abuse marijuana, which provides short-term relief but ultimately exacerbates his anxiety and dysfunction.

Moderate Personality Disorder

In Moderate Personality Disorder, multiple areas of functioning (e.g., stability and coherence of identity, self-worth, and self-direction) are affected to some degree. There are marked problems in most interpersonal relationships and the performance of most expected social and occupational roles is compromised to some degree. Relationships are likely to be characterised by conflict, avoidance, withdrawal, or extreme dependency (e.g., few friendships maintained, persistent conflict in work relationships causing occupational problems, romantic relationships characterised by serious disruption or inappropriate submissiveness). Moderate Personality Disorder is sometimes associated with harm to self or others. It is associated with marked impairment in personal, family, social, educational, occupational, or other important areas of functioning, although functioning in circumscribed areas may be maintained.

In Moderate Personality Disorder, the individual's sense of self may become particularly incoherent in times of crises. The individual has considerable difficulty maintaining positive self-esteem or, alternatively, has an unrealistically positive self-view that is not modified by evidence to the contrary. The individual exhibits poor emotion regulation in the face of setbacks, often becoming highly upset and giving up easily, which eventually compromises self-direction. Alternatively, the individual may persist unreasonably in pursuit of goals that have no chance of success. The individual may exhibit little genuine interest in, or efforts towards, sustained employment. Major limitations in the ability to understand and appreciate others' perspectives hinder developing close and mutually satisfying relationships. There are persistent problems in those relationships that do exist, which may be characterised by frequent, serious, and volatile conflicts, or be significantly unbalanced (e.g., the individual is highly dominant or overly compliant). Under stress, there are marked distortions in the individual's situational and interpersonal appraisals, which may involve mild dissociative states or psychotic-like beliefs or perceptions (e.g., paranoid ideas). The next two case examples are meant to illustrate how a Moderate Personality Disorder may manifest and are by no means exhaustive of the variation found in clinical settings.

Case: Eva

Eva is a 40-year-old single mum of two sons aged 17 and 21 years from two different relationships. The father of her youngest son is serving a sentence for a brutal crime and Eva is in frequent contact with him, transferring money to him every month despite her own financial struggles. The man threatens her not to file for divorce or to stop sending him money. Although the situation pains her, it also gives her a sense of security to fantasise about the day he returns from prison, and it will be the two of them forever.

Throughout her life, Eva has felt unsure of who she was and what her life was meant to be. She is very self-sacrificing towards her grown-up children, often sending them money. Her 21-year-old son takes advantage of her and, despite having a full-time job, he still complains that she does not support him enough financially. Eva sometimes punishes herself by "falling" down the stairs, eating only very unhealthy food, and at other times starving herself.

This general dynamic seems to be almost a repetition of some experiences she had as a child with her mentally disturbed mother, who ran a brothel in their home. Eva helped out in her mum's business from a young age. Despite this, she managed to do well in school and college, socially and academically, while dealing with the abuse that took place in her home the best she could. She left home as a teenager and has had a series of jobs and partners without really settling in. For most of her life, she has suffered from anxiety and feelings of emptiness and despair.

When Eva begins group therapy at a psychiatric hospital, she has very little trust in the therapists and other group members. Over time, she comes to idealise the therapist as a kind of saviour, although this sometimes alternates with a perception of the therapist as a traitor who will ultimately let her down. She is often over-involved in the personal problems of her fellow patients and feels a need to rescue them, partly as a distraction from her own problems. This is initially perceived as positive by her fellow patients but, over time, it starts to annoy them that she shows so little of her own vulnerability. Eventually, she feels that no one in the group likes her.

Case: Tristan

Tristan is a 50-year-old man who, until recently, was a highly competent employee in an administrative job. Since his early youth, he has been preoccupied with perfection and achievement. At times his behaviour is excessive, pedantic, and stubborn. He always has the "right" solution to challenges and feels completely comfortable talking about and solving complicated problems, regardless of his actual expertise in the field. However, when he comes into contact with other highly competent people, he becomes quiet, inhibited, and uncomfortable.

Usually feeling superior and entitled at work, Tristan can become spiteful and perfidious when his value and achievements are not recognised by others. However, he is very pleasing and accommodating to his superiors. Tristan has often been unwilling to cooperate or delegate "important" tasks unless others agree to exactly his way of doing things.

Colleagues and other people describe him as aggressive, sensitive, emotionally unbalanced, controlling, domineering, petty, and arrogant. A former colleague called Tristan a "narcissistic control freak," whereas Tristan referred to that colleague as being "weak and unintelligent." Several former colleagues have apparently resigned because of him, at least two of them after long-term sick leave and referrals to a psychologist.

Tristan has not been able to maintain steady employment due to conflicts with colleagues and managers, or maintain close relationships outside the workplace. According to him, it has always been his own decision to quit various jobs throughout his career, typically when he had realised that his colleagues were too incompetent and that his employers were not up to the task of managing someone with his particular skills. But, after a recent case involving the human resource department, Tristan was formally dismissed before he realised what was going on.

This happened shortly after his girlfriend left him. As a result, he no longer had any professional status or close personal relationships. It was difficult for him to get a new job due to the many job changes on his CV, and his extravagant lifestyle has put him under financial pressure. Tristan felt deep shame and experienced a massive emotional trauma that has been hidden for decades under a veneer of superiority and competence. One night, the police found him walking on a bridge with apparent suicidal intent and he was taken to a psychiatric emergency room.

Severe Personality Disorder

In Severe Personality Disorder, multiple areas of functioning are severely affected. For example, the sense of self may be so unstable that individuals report not having a sense of who they are or so rigid that they refuse to participate in any but an extremely narrow range of situations. The self-view may be characterised by self-contempt or be grandiose or highly eccentric. Problems in interpersonal functioning seriously affect virtually all relationships, and the ability and willingness to perform expected social and occupational roles are severely compromised or absent. Specific manifestations of personality disturbances at this level are severe and affect most, if not all, areas of personality functioning. Severe Personality Disorder is often associated with harm to self or others and with severe impairment in all or nearly all areas of life, including personal, family, social, educational, occupational, and other important areas of functioning.

In Severe Personality Disorder, the person's self-view is very unrealistic and typically highly unstable or contradictory, and the individual is largely unable to set and pursue realistic goals. There is typically serious difficulty with regulation of self-esteem, emotional experience and expression, and impulse control, as well as other aspects of behaviour (e.g., perseveration, indecision). The individual's interpersonal relationships, if any, lack mutuality, are shallow, extremely one-sided, unstable, or highly conflictual, often to the point of violence. Family relationships are absent (despite having living relatives) or marred by significant conflict. The individual has extreme difficulty acknowledging difficult or unwanted emotions (e.g., does not recognise or acknowledge experiencing anger, sadness, or other emotions). The individual is unwilling or unable to sustain regular work due to lack of interest or effort, poor performance (e.g., failure to complete assignments or perform expected roles, unreliability), interpersonal difficulties, or inappropriate behaviour (e.g., fits of temper, insubordination). Under stress, there are extreme distortions in the individual's situational and interpersonal appraisals (i.e., reality testing; see further definition in Chapter 3), which often involve dissociative states or psychotic-like beliefs or perceptions (e.g., extreme paranoid reactions). The next two case examples are intended to illustrate how a Severe Personality Disorder can manifest itself and are by no means exhaustive of the variation found in clinical settings.

Case: Edith

Edith is a 27-year-old socially isolated woman with a history of several serious suicide attempts that have resulted in repeated hospitalisations, failed medication attempts, and interrupted psychotherapy sessions. Since she was around 13 years old, her life has been complicated by an Eating Disorder, anxiety attacks, depression, Obesssive-Compulsive Disorder, cannabis abuse, dangerous self-harm, and unstable relationships.

Throughout her childhood, Edith was verbally, physically, and sexually abused by her stepfather and an uncle, while being neglected by her mother. She has never known her biological father. When she feels under a lot of pressure and emotionally upset, Edith hears a voice telling her that she is a useless person and should punish herself, which is accompanied by feelings of emptiness and out-of-body sensations. Although she has some insight into the meaning of the voices, such episodes often result in self-harm and suicide attempts. Stressful interpersonal situations can also cause delusional-like perceptions that people around her are ganging up on her.

In recent years, her excessive distrust of other people has taken a toll on her social network. As a young adult, Edith had various boyfriends from the criminal world who sexually abused her and to whom she submitted for fear of abandonment. She has always struggled to figure out who she is and what to do with her life. Even in the best of times, she has felt a bit like a chameleon, always adapting to other people's value systems and beliefs without ever finding out who the real Edith is.

Case: Thor

Thor is a 34-year-old man who is in prison after multiple counts of rape and two counts of assault resulting in death. A forensic mental health assessment concluded that he was dangerous to his surroundings, and he was sentenced to custody.

Thor appears intelligent, handsome, charming, and confident. He has manipulated his victims by presenting himself as a fascinating and charismatic gentleman. But beneath this surface, Thor lived as a parasitic and opportunistic deceiver whose primary means of relating to others was exploitation. For example, he repeatedly took advantage of a lonely woman who allowed him to stay in her home.

Thor regularly had affairs with other women, sometimes involving rape and brutality if they resisted participating in the sexual activity he felt entitled to have with them. When asked, Thor says that he feels he did the women a favour because he was convinced that it is every woman's secret dream to have sex with a man like him.

Thor feels justified in taking money, credit cards, and other valuable possessions from his victims. He never feels remorse or any concern for them, but rather seems proud of all he has accomplished, while smilingly referring to himself as something of a "pick-up artist."

Chapter 5

Trait Domains

In addition to the basic classification of severity, as mentioned, ICD-11 also allows for a more detailed and individualised description of personality dysfunction through the specification of one or more trait domains. The specific trait domains (and their characteristics) can be used to portray the unique pattern of personality traits or styles that contribute to the overall personality dysfunction. Clinicians may think of these five trait domains, which are grounded in the scientific literature on personality (Mulder et al., 2011; Widiger & Crego, 2019; Widiger & Simonsen, 2005), as entities that are replacing the stylistic features of traditional Personality Disorder types (see Appendix B). These specifiers are thus used to describe individual stylistic features of the Personality Disorder or sub-diagnostic Personality Difficulty. Table 5.1 gives abbreviated descriptions of these trait domains.

Table 5.1 Abbreviated descriptions of trait domains

Negative Affectivity	Experiences a broad range of negative emotions with a frequency and intensity out of proportion to the situation, which may involve emotional lability and poor emotion regulation, negativistic attitudes, low self-esteem and self-confidence, and mistrustfulness.
Detachment	Maintains interpersonal distance (social detachment) and emotional distance (emotional detachment), which may include avoidance of social interactions, lack of friendships, avoidance of intimacy, as well as limited emotional expression and experience and being emotionally reserved and aloof.
Dissociality	Disregards the rights and feelings of others, encompassing both self-centredness (e.g., sense of entitlement, expectation of others' admiration, positive or negative attention-seeking behaviours) and lack of empathy (i.e., callous about whether one's actions hurt others, being manipulative and mean).

Table 5.1   Continued

Disinhibition	Acts rashly based on immediate external or internal stimuli (i.e., sensations, emotions, thoughts), without consideration of potential negative consequences. Common manifestations are impulsivity, distractibility, irresponsibility, recklessness, and lack of planning.
Anankastia	A narrow focus on one's rigid standard of perfection and of right and wrong, and on controlling one's own and others' behaviour and controlling situations to ensure conformity to these standards.

Specifiers for trait domains are relevant because they provide an understanding of individual triggers and stressors that can induce and amplify problems in the person (Bach & Presnall-Shvorin, 2020). Specifiers can point to how we best interact with and establish a therapeutic relationship with the patient. For example, it makes a significant difference in treatment whether a Personality Disorder is expressed as excessively anxious and avoidant (trait domains of Negative Affectivity and Detachment) or highly self-centred and reckless (trait domains of Dissociality and Disinhibition). These two different expressions reflect different forms of personality dysfunction and can form the basis for different approaches to clinical management.

It is possible to code as many trait domains as necessary to describe the individual and their typical difficulties. Interpretation of combined trait domains will usually say more about the person than separate trait domains on their own. For example, two individuals who are both characterised by Negative Affectivity may have significant characteristics in common, including emotional lability. However, one person has a combination with Detachment (e.g., internalised anger, avoidance, and self-blame), while the other has a combination with Dissociality (e.g., externalised anger, confrontation, and blaming others). Furthermore, the number or complexity of predominant domains often reflects the overall severity of the disorder. A Severe Personality Disorder is therefore usually characterised by multiple predominant trait domains, whereas a Mild Personality Disorder may be associated with only one predominant trait domain. However, in some cases, a patient may have a Severe Personality Disorder and only manifest a single prominent trait (such as Dissociality) that may pose serious danger to others. Table 5.2 shows examples of how trait domains can manifest differently depending on severity.

Table 5.2 Trait domains at different levels of severity

	Negative affectivity	Detachment	Dissociality	Disinhibition	Anankastia
None	Naturally sensitive with healthy regulation and experience of a wide range of emotions.	Generally, thrives best in their own company, but appreciates a few good, stable friends and feels like a valued member of the community.	Confident, courageous, and decisive, but generally able to put themselves in the shoes of others without hurting or offending anyone. Strives for cooperation and the common good.	Comes up with new useful ideas, is spontaneous and takes risks in life, but is able to cooperate and respect the rules, demands, and order of others.	Tidy, organised, competent, and ambitious, but able to flexibly respond to others' ideas and sometimes give themselves a break.
Personality Difficulty	Strong emotions can cause some reduction in self-esteem, integrity, and well-being.	Has some friendships that are not really that deep or satisfying. Limits emotional expression or withdraws if they lead to conflict or intense emotions.	Personal standards can be quite self-centred with a slightly reduced ability to respect or appreciate the feelings of others. Other people may be perceived as oversensitive.	Able to act and take risks adaptively, but sometimes a little too risky or reckless. May appear impatient, distracted, or easily bored.	Certain standards in relation to oneself or others can inhibit co-operation and limit aspects of a fulfilling life.

Table 5.2 Continued

	Negative affectivity	Detachment	Dissociality	Disinhibition	Anankastia
Mild Personality Disorder	Threats to self-esteem can elicit strong emotions, and fear of failure can cause inhibition in achieving goals.	Has few relationships outside of family and little interpersonal interest. Solo activity is common. Emotionally inhibited and socially withdrawn.	Entitled, uncaring, self-centred, and mostly concerned with personal gain. Expects to be admired by others.	Personal standards are unreasonably low (e.g., sloppy, careless). Acts on impulse in an often disruptive manner.	Personal standards become unreasonable and rigid, and the importance of productivity can become over-emphasised.
Moderate Personality Disorder	Rapidly changing emotions, chronic sadness or anxiety with fragile self-esteem, shame, and interpersonal sensitivity.	Has only some superficial acquaintances outside family and often seems to be disconnected and indifferent to interpersonal exchanges. Generally, avoids activities with others.	Self-aggrandising, hostile, exploitative, and manipulative with some risk of abusing or harming others.	Risky behaviour and impulsivity regardless of negative consequences for self or others. Sometimes with risk of harm to self or others.	Excessive and rigid standards cause problems collaborating with others and compromise authenticity and social life.
Severe Personality Disorder	Constant self-hatred and a corresponding distrust of others. Hatred and anger can be dominant emotional states. Risk of self-harm.	Almost always avoids other people with deep interpersonal distance, emotional withdrawal, lack of interest, and sometimes distrust.	Callous, cunning, manipulative, cruel, and only respect their own rules. Serious risk of intentionally harming others.	Reckless and impulsive behaviour without considering the harmful consequences for self and others. Pronounced risk of harm to self or others.	Extreme and overly rigid standards that compromise the ability to live with other people, achieve goals, and have a fulfilling life.

Negative Affectivity

The trait domain of Negative Affectivity contains features that are probably known to many as Neuroticism according to the five-factor model of personality (McCrae, 1991), but with a greater emphasis on pathological trait expressions such as anger and hostility instead of irritability. This domain thus includes the tendency to experience negative emotions in a broad sense. Here, we highlight key characteristics of Negative Affectivity, which include emotionality out of proportion to the situation, lability and poor emotion regulation, negativistic attitudes, low self-esteem and self-confidence, and distrust. It should be emphasised that the manifestation of specific negative emotions depends mainly on the other trait domains, including their level of severity. For example, people with high levels of Dissociality are more likely to experience externalising negative emotions (anger, hostility, contempt), while people with high levels of Detachment are more likely to experience internalising negative emotions (anxiety, depression, pessimism, guilt).

- *Negative emotions with a frequency and intensity that is disproportionate to the situation*
  - Fear and anxiety
  - Worry
  - Depression
  - Vulnerability
  - Anger
  - Hostility
  - Guilt
  - Shame
- *Emotional lability and poor emotion regulation*
  - Over-reactive to both your own negative beliefs and external events
  - May become upset as a result of their own thought processes, such as rumination over their own shortcomings or past mistakes, over real or perceived threats, slights or insults, or potential future problems
  - Over-reactive to external threats or criticism as well as problems and setbacks
  - Low frustration tolerance and easily (visibly) emotionally affected by even small problems
  - Often experience and display multiple emotions simultaneously or fluctuate between a range of emotions within a short period of time
  - Difficulty regaining composure and need to seek support from others or leave the situation to find peace

- *Negativistic attitudes*
  - Typically reject other people's suggestions or advice, claiming it will be too complicated or difficult to follow
  - Perceives that other people's suggestions will not lead to desired results or may even lead to negative consequences
  - Tend to blame others or themselves for problems or poor performance
- *Low self-esteem and confidence*
  - Exhibit low self-esteem and confidence in a variety of ways
  - Avoids situations and activities that, despite evidence to the contrary, are deemed too difficult (intellectually, physically, socially, interpersonally, emotionally, etc.)
  - Dependency, which can manifest as frequent reliance on others for advice, guidance, and other forms of help
  - Envy of others' abilities and signs of success
  - With very low self-esteem, the person may perceive themselves as useless, living a worthless life, and unable to achieve anything of value, which may be accompanied by suicidal thoughts or behaviour
- *Distrust*
  - Suspicion that others have negative intentions, and that neutral or even well-intentioned remarks and positive behaviours are hidden threats, slights, or insults
  - Tendency to hold grudges and not being able to forgive even for a long time
  - Bitterness and cynicism (e.g., a belief that "the system is rotten and corrupt")

Detachment

This trait domain describes the tendency to distance oneself from other people and one's own emotional life. The key characteristics of this domain are listed, which include social and emotional withdrawal.

- *Social Detachment*
  - Avoiding social interactions
  - Lack of friendships
  - Avoiding proximity
  - Lack of enjoyment in social interactions
  - Avoids all forms of social contact and social situations as much as possible
  - Engages in little or no small talk, even when others initiate it (e.g., at the supermarket checkout)

- Seek employment that does not involve interaction with others and even turn down a promotion if it will lead to more social interaction
- Have few or no friendships or even casual acquaintances
- Interaction with family members tends to be minimal and superficial
- Rarely, if ever, involved in intimate relationships and show reduced interest in sexual relationships
- *Emotional Detachment*
  - Reservation, unapproachability, and limited emotional expression and experience
  - Keep to themselves as much as possible, even in situations where socialising is unavoidable
  - Is typically reserved, withdrawn, and responds only briefly to direct attempts at social interaction, including responding in ways that discourage further conversation
  - Emotional numbness, both verbal and non-verbal
  - Does not talk about feelings and is difficult to read emotionally
  - In extreme cases, the emotional experience itself is missing
  - Reacts neither to negative nor positive events and has limited capacity for pleasure and enjoyment

Dissociality

Here, we highlight key characteristics of Dissociality, which include self-centredness and lack of empathy. It should be emphasised that these characteristics can be both active (e.g., attention-seeking behaviour) and passive (e.g., an expectation of others' admiration). It should also be emphasised that people with predominant Dissociality usually have an intact cognitive understanding of other people's emotions, but just do not care as much about those emotions. On this basis, they may be inclined to use a cognitive understanding to ultimately exploit others (e.g., cold mentalisation).

- *Self-centredness*
  - A perception of special status and an expectation of admiration from others
  - Self-concept and behaviours are based on deserving whatever they desire, feel entitled to take precedence over others, and that this should be obvious to everyone
  - Attention-seeking behaviour to ensure being the centre of attention and exhibit negative behaviour (e.g., anger, tantrums, and belittling others) when this admiration and attention is missing

- Conviction of possessing many admirable. qualities and outstanding achievements and being almost destined to achieve great things and the admiration of others
- Indifference to the fact that other people have as much value as you do
- Preoccupation with own needs, wants, and well-being while ignoring the needs, wants, and well-being of others
- *Lack of empathy*
  - Indifference to whether their actions are an inconvenience or hurt others in any way (e.g., emotionally, socially, financially, physically)
  - Deceptive, manipulative, and exploitative
  - Malice and physical aggression can turn violent at the slightest, perhaps imagined, provocation
  - Cynicism towards other people's suffering
  - Recklessness and carelessness in the pursuit of personal goals
  - May in some cases feel pleasure in causing pain and harm (i.e., sadism)

Disinhibition

This trait domain describes the tendency to act rashly based on immediate external or internal stimuli (i.e., sensations, emotions, thoughts) without regard for potential negative consequences. We highlight key characteristics of this domain, which include aspects of impulsivity, distractibility, irresponsibility, risk-taking behaviour, and lack of planning.

- *Impulsivity*
  - Tendency to act rashly based on whatever appears attractive in the moment, without consideration of negative consequences for oneself or others, including physical danger
  - Difficulty delaying rewards or gratification and tends to seek out immediately available, short-term pleasures or potential gains
  - Associated with, for example, drug abuse, gambling, and impulsive sexual activity
- *Distractibility*
  - Have difficulty staying focused on important and necessary tasks that require sustained effort
  - Become easily bored or frustrated with difficult, routine, or lengthy tasks
  - Easily distracted by extraneous stimuli such as other people's conversations
  - Difficulty staying focused and working persistently on tasks and therefore tends to scan the environment for more enjoyable opportunities, even in the absence of distractions

- *Irresponsibility*
  - Unreliability and lack of accountability for their actions
  - Often do not get work tasks or chores done
  - Fails to meet deadlines, commitments, and promises, and misses or fails to attend appointments due to more attractive opportunities or sudden impulses
- *Recklessness*
  - Lacks an appropriate sense of caution
  - Tend to overestimate their own abilities and therefore often do things that are beyond their skill level without considering potential safety risks
  - May be involved in reckless driving or dangerous sports or engaging in other activities that endanger themselves or others without adequate preparation or training
- *Lack of planning*
  - Prefers spontaneous over planned activities and leaves options open should a more attractive opportunity arise
  - Tends to focus on immediate feelings, sensations, and thoughts with relatively little attention paid to long-term or even short-term goals
  - Rarely follows through with plans
  - Are seldom able to reach long-term goals, and often fail to achieve even short-term goals

Anankastia

Here, we highlight key characteristics of Anankastia, which include aspects of perfectionism as well as emotional and behavioural constraint.

- *Perfectionism*
  - Concern with social rules, obligations, and norms of right and wrong
  - Scrupulous attention to details, rigid and systematic daily routines, excessive scheduling and planning, and an emphasis on organisation, orderliness, and neatness
  - Very clear and detailed personal sense of perfection and imperfection that also extends beyond community standards to encompass the individual's idiosyncratic notions of what is perfect and right
  - Strongly believes that everyone should follow all rules exactly and meet all obligations
  - May redo the work of others because it does not meet their perfectionistic standards

–   Have difficulties in interpersonal relationships because they hold oth-
     ers to the same standards as themselves and are inflexible in their views
- *Emotional and behavioural constraint*
  –   Manifests in rigid control over emotional expression, stubbornness and
       inflexibility, risk avoidance, perseveration, and deliberativeness
  –   Exercises tight control over their own emotional expressions and disap-
       proves of others' display of emotion
  –   Lacks flexibility and spontaneity
  –   Stubbornly insist on following set schedules and adhering to plans
  –   Risk avoidance includes both refusal to engage in risky activities and a
       more general over-concern about avoiding potential negative conse-
       quences of any activity
  –   Often perseveres and has difficulty disengaging from tasks because they
       are perceived as not yet perfect down to the last detail
  –   Are highly deliberative and have difficulty making decisions due to con-
       cern that they have not considered all possible aspects and alternatives
       to ensure that the right decision is made

How Traits Contribute To Personality Dysfunction

The ICD-11 explicitly states that the five trait domains describe the characteristics of the individual's personality that are most prominent and that contribute to personality disturbance (World Health Organization, 2024, p. 553).
Table 5.3 presents a summary of how the five trait domains may contribute
to this disturbance according to aspects of the self and interpersonal functioning as well as emotional, cognitive, and behavioral manifestations.

Borderline Pattern Specifier

ICD-11 includes the option of specifying a borderline pattern, primarily out of
consideration for the extensive amount of psychotherapy literature and national
guidelines that have been developed over the past 30 years with a focus on this
diagnosis (Reed, 2018; Storebø et al., 2020). At the same time, the scientific literature recognises and broadly agrees that there is significant overlap between
the borderline pattern and the information contained in the definition of global
Personality Disorder severity and the specified trait domains (e.g., Clark et al.,
2018; Gutiérrez, Aluja, Ruiz Rodríguez et al., 2023; Sharp, 2018).

Table 5.3.   Summary of how trait domains may contribute to aspects of personality disturbance

	Self	Interpersonal	Emotional	Cognitive	Behavioural
Negative affectivity	Low self-esteem and goal-inhibition due to anxiousness or feelings of inadequacy.	Over-reliant on others for advice, direction, help, and emotion regulation. Sometimes mistrustful and envious of others' abilities and indicators of success.	Over-reactive to internal and external emotional stimuli including vacillation among a range of negative emotions in a short period of time.	Ruminative cognitive style and difficulty making decisions in situations of uncertainty. Rigid beliefs about being worthless and that others are being critical or rejecting.	Easily become visibly upset, which may result in harm to self or others, and sometimes they must leave the situation to calm down.
Detachment	Self-direction is compromised by lack of personal drive as well as refusal of occupation that involves social interaction.	Social detachment and avoidance of social interactions, lack of friendships, and avoidance of intimacy.	Emotionally underreactive and detached. Non-reactive to either negative or positive events, with a limited capacity for enjoyment	Decision making characterized by disinterest, avoidance or lack of pleasure.	Social withdrawal and expressive suppression in stressful situations. Otherwise, their behaviour does not reveal what they might be feeling or thinking.

Table 5.3. Continued

	Self	Interpersonal	Emotional	Cognitive	Behavioural
Dissociality	Sense of grandiosity with goal setting that is solely based on personal satisfaction.	Disregard rights and feelings of others, lack of empathy, and exploits others.	Over-reactive in terms of temper tantrums and under-reactive in terms of callousness and unemotionality.	Fixed beliefs about being entitled and superior while other people do not matter.	Attention seeking, hostile, and sometimes physically aggressive behaviours.
Disinhibition	Lack self-direction with respect to long-term goals and tend to overestimate their own abilities in risky situations.	Do not follow through on commitments and promises, and may put others in danger (e.g., physically or financially)	Tendency to focus on and express immediate feelings.	Distractibility and poor decision making based on what is compelling at the moment.	Behaviourally under-controlled in terms of reckless and risk taking behaviours with lack of planning.
Anankastia	Identity is overly fixed on productive roles with rigid and uncompromising self-directedness.	Interpersonal conflicts because they hold others to the same standards as themselves, while they disapprove of others' displays of emotion.	Rigid control over emotional expression including joy, fun, and other unproductive aspects.	A belief system characterized by rigid and inflexible ideas of perfection and rules.	Behaviourally over-controlled in terms of risk avoidance, perfectionism, and lack of spontaneity.

It should be emphasised that the borderline pattern is an additional specifier and not an actual diagnosis. In any case, clinicians must first and foremost determine whether a Personality Disorder is present, then its severity, and, if desired, one or more trait domains can then be coded with the possibility of also indicating a borderline pattern. The classification of severity and coding of trait domains thus precedes any coding of a borderline pattern. Tables 5.4 and 5.5 illustrate how individuals with a borderline pattern may be characterized according to aspects of personality functioning and the three severity levels, where Mild Personality Disorder would capture subthreshold borderline features. We also refer to Appendix B for a portrayal of borderline features by means of ICD-11 aspects of personality functioning and trait domains.

The borderline pattern specifier can be applied to individuals whose personality disturbances are characterised by a pervasive pattern of instability in interpersonal relationships, self-image, affects, and marked impulsivity, as indicated by five (or more) of the following features (World Health Organisation, 2024, p. 564).

- Frantic efforts to avoid real or imagined abandonment.
- A pattern of unstable and intense interpersonal relationships, which may be characterised by vacillations between idealisation and devaluation, typically associated with both strong desire for, and fear of, closeness and intimacy.
- Identity disturbance, manifested in markedly and persistently unstable self-view or sense of self.
- A tendency to act rashly in states of high negative affect, leading to potentially self-damaging behaviours (e.g., risky sexual behaviour, reckless driving, excessive alcohol or substance use, binge eating).
- Recurrent episodes of self-harm (e.g., suicide attempts or gestures, self-mutilation).
- Emotional instability due to marked reactivity of mood. Fluctuations of mood may be triggered either internally (e.g., by one's own thoughts) or by external events. As a consequence, the individual experiences intense dysphoric mood states, which typically last for a few hours, but may last up to several days.
- Chronic feelings of emptiness.
- Inappropriate intense anger or difficulty controlling anger manifested in frequent displays of temper (e.g., yelling or screaming, throwing or breaking things, getting into physical fights).
- Transient dissociative symptoms or psychotic-like features (e.g., brief hallucinations, paranoia) in situations of high affective arousal.

Other manifestations of the borderline pattern, not all of which may occur in the person at the same time, include the following.

- A view of the self as inadequate, bad, guilty, disgusting, and contemptible.
- An experience of the self as profoundly different and isolated from other people; a painful sense of alienation and pervasive loneliness.
- Proneness to rejection hypersensitivity, problems in establishing and maintaining consistent and appropriate levels of trust in interpersonal relationships, frequent misinterpretation of social signals.

Table 5.4   Borderline pattern features captured by aspects of personality functioning

Personality functioning		
Aspects of the self	**Interpersonal functioning**	
• Identity disturbance • A negative view of the self • An experience of the self as profoundly different and isolated	• Frantic efforts to avoid abandonment • Unstable and intense relationships • Proneness to rejection hypersensitivity • Problems with interpersonal trust	
Manifestations		
Emotional	**Cognitive**	**Behaviour**
• Emotional instability • Chronic feelings of emptiness • Inappropriate intense anger	• Dissociative or psychotic-like features • Misinterpretation of social signals	• Acts rashly in states of high negative affect • Recurrent episodes of self-harm
Global psychosocial impairment and/or distress		
Personal, family, social, educational, employment or other significant functioning		

Table 5.5   Example of what a borderline pattern might look like at three different severity levels according to the ICD-11 diagnostic classification

Mild	• Sense of self may be somewhat contradictory • Weak ability to set appropriate goals and to work towards them • Relationships characterised by intermittent or frequent minor conflicts that are not so severe that they cause serious disruption • Typically not associated with substantial harm to self or others • Under stress, there may be some distortions in the individual's situational and interpersonal appraisals, but reality testing typically remains intact. (e.g., four to five out of nine borderline features)
Moderate	• Sense of self may become incoherent, particularly in times of crisis • Often becoming highly upset and giving up goals easily • Relationships characterised by frequent, serious, and volatile conflict • Sometimes associated with harm to self or others • Under stress, there may be mild dissociative states or psychotic-like beliefs or perceptions (e.g., paranoid ideas) (e.g., five to seven out of nine borderline features)
Severe	• Self-view is very unrealistic and typically highly unstable or contradictory • Largely unable to set and pursue realistic goals • Relationships are highly conflictual, often to the point of violence • Often associated with harm to self or others • Under stress, there are often dissociative states or psychotic-like beliefs or perceptions (e.g., extreme paranoid reactions) (e.g., seven to nine out of nine borderline features)

Chapter 6

Clinical Decision Making and Treatment

In this chapter, we will first present suggestions on how the severity of a Personality Disorder in general can guide clinical decisions and treatment management. Subsequently, we will review how trait domains and their combinations can guide both the treatment of, and the way we interact with, patients.

Severity and Clinical Decisions

Overall, as mentioned earlier, see Allport (1937), the severity of personality dysfunction relates to what the personality *does* (i.e., how we manage ourselves in relation to others), which can often also change or vary across time and situation. Therefore, treatment focuses on personality functioning or severity and less on the personality traits that have a higher degree of stability and make up what personality *is* (i.e., our stylistic disposition). Adapting treatment to what personality *does* and what personality *is* therefore also are two different things (Bach, 2020; Bach & Simonsen, 2021; Bach & Tracy, 2022; Kiel, Hopwood et al., 2024). In contrast to personality traits and traditional Personality Disorder types, the global dimension of personality functioning appears to capture core vulnerabilities of personality-disordered patients that are related to future functioning and symptom severity (Weekers et al., 2024).

In particular, severity provides the clinician with important information about the expected level of risk and treatment prognosis. Thus, harm to self and others is rare in individuals with Personality Difficulty and Mild Personality Disorder, while the risk of harm to self and others is relatively frequent in Severe Personality Disorder. For example, the risk of severe self-harm or suicide attempts means that, in most cases, the clinician should pay extra attention to developing a crisis management plan with the patient (Moselli et al., 2023). The risk level also relates to violence and harm to others (Allen & Links, 2012). A comprehensive systematic review of studies of prison inmates found that a total of 65% had a Personality Disorder and, of these, approximately 46% had a diagnosis of Antisocial Personality Disorder (Fazel & Danesh, 2002). It is anticipated that future research based on the ICD-11 classification of Personality Disorder will contribute to more accurate description and prediction in areas such as forensic settings (Carroll et al., 2022; Hopwood & Sellbom, 2013).

In relation to treatment prognosis, the determination of severity can especially help the clinician to align expectations for treatment alliance and treatment progression (Bach & Simonsen, 2021). The treatment alliance in Personality Disorders is often different from treatment for other mental disorders (Bender, 2005). This is because personality dysfunction and its manifestations often manifest in the relationship with the therapist or treatment provider. In the treatment of Personality Difficulty and Mild Personality Disorder, there will typically be no significant alliance problems, while non-alliance and alliance ruptures will be more frequent as severity of dysfunction increases. With respect to prognosis and treatment progression, research indicates that patients with lower personality functioning are more inclined to drop-out of therapy (Kiel, Hopwood et al., 2024). It might seem obvious that patients with the most severe level of dysfunction and the most pronounced trust issues are also those with the poorest treatment alliance, which naturally leads to higher risk of drop-out. See Table 6.1 for examples of how personality functioning can affect the alliance with the therapist.

Table 6.1 Possible effect of personality dysfunction on the alliance with a therapist

Personality dysfunction and manifestation	Effect on alliance
Incoherent and unstable identity	Often leads to ambiguity and confusion on the part of the practitioner, which can spur further disorganisation of personality functioning
Difficulty recognising own attributes, strengths, and limitations	Leads to confusion and possible disagreement about the goals and tasks of the treatment
Lack of ability to understand and appreciate the perspectives of others	Leads to misunderstandings and often challenges the emotional bond with the therapist
Tendency to be emotionally over- or underreactive	Often leads to over- or underresponsiveness of the clinician depending on their own personality functioning

Table 6.1   Continued

Personality dysfunction and manifestation	Effect on alliance
Problems recognising and acknowledging difficult or unwanted emotions in themselves	Often leads to misunderstandings, as the therapist may attribute feelings to the person that they do not feel or recognise
Lack of stability and flexibility in beliefs	Often leads to a sense of being stuck that is often frustrating for the practitioner; alternatively, beliefs can be so fluid and malleable that treatment goals and tasks are constantly shifting
Inappropriate behavioural responses to intense emotions and stressful circumstances	Risk of self-harm or aggression can paralyse the alliance and compromise an authentic therapeutic relationship

General Treatment Principles for Personality Disorder

Knowledge of how to treat Borderline Personality Disorder can be used to distil some key principles that address personality functioning in general, and in some cases can guide how treatment varies depending on whether the disorder is mild, moderate, or severe. Hopwood (2018) and Bateman and colleagues (2015) have reviewed the treatment literature and have come up with the five transtheoretical principles for effective treatment of Personality Disorder, which are presented in Box 6.1 and then elaborated on.

Box 6.1
Transtheoretical principles for effective treatment of Personality Disorder

1. The higher the severity, the more important it is to have a structured approach to treatment.
2. Focus on promoting and clarifying agency, that is, personal responsibility in treatment (i.e., self-direction and decision-making).
3. Focus on fostering the connection between emotions, events, and actions.
4. Focus on the therapist role and an appropriate activity level.
5. Focus on opportunities for supervision.

---

1. *The higher the severity, the more important it is to have a structured approach to treatment.* People with Severe Personality Disorder are affected in a wide range of areas (work, relationships, etc.). At the same time, they also struggle with the personality resources that are available to manage themselves in these areas. Without a certain structure to prioritise the problems and a consistent model of intervention, we risk that treatment goes in many directions, ultimately wearing away faith in more lasting and substantial personality changes. Manualised therapies are examples of how a higher degree of structure can be achieved in the treatment of moderate to severe Personality Disorders. However, in some cases, patients with high severity may find that they may need to be supported in specific and more circumscribed goals in types of treatment that cannot be described as manualised or highly structured. This type of treatment, which is probably rather prevalent in community mental health services, is an area with very sparse research (Ledden et al., 2022).

2. *Focus on promoting and clarifying agency, that is, personal responsibility in treatment.* Contrary to the first principle, it will not necessarily be the case that higher severity implies a greater focus on agency. Instead, it can be said that, in almost all cases, the issue of ownership, role allocation, etc., will become relevant in the treatment of people with Personality Disorder. The concrete expression will often be influenced by specific personality traits but, regardless, the understanding of one's own role in treatment will almost always come into play in a more complicated way than in the treatment of other disorders.

3. *Focus on promoting the connection between emotions, events, and actions.* Whether it is Mild, Moderate, or Severe Personality Disorder, treatment will focus on the relationship between emotions and situations. In mild cases, this will often involve a lack of connection to certain emotions (e.g., anger) in certain types of situations or relationships, while, in severe cases, the person cannot be made to recognise certain unwanted emotions at all and is often severely emotionally dysregulated. A characteristic feature of all evidence-based psychotherapies for Borderline Personality Disorder is that the manuals contain specific interventions that work to strengthen the person's ability to associate emotions with events/actions.

4. *Focus on the therapist's role and an appropriate level of activity.* Evidence-based forms of psychotherapy are characterised by the therapist being quite active and engaged in the treatment process. Regardless of the specific approach, therapists will almost invariably feel pressured in a certain direction in their role as a therapist when working with people with Personality Disorders. For example, a study by Folmo and colleagues (2021) showed that people with more Severe Personality Disorder, characterised by dis-

trust, benefited most from treatment when the therapist was able to maintain a straightforward and transparent communication style. In cases where treatment outcomes were poor, this was mainly due to the fact that, over time, distrustful patients often experienced increasing disagreement with their therapists about therapy tasks.

5. *Focus on opportunities for supervision and guidance.* In continuation of the fourth principle regarding the role of the therapist, all of the evidence-based psychotherapies require opportunities for supervision in order to help the therapist help the patient.

While the overarching principles for supervision are largely based on what therapists should be aware of when working with people with Personality Disorder, another general approach has focused more on how treatment can be guided by adapting to different areas of personality dysfunction (Clarkin et al., 2015). This model focuses on four areas of dysfunction: symptom distress, emotion regulation, relational functioning, and self-functioning. The different evidence-based treatments will often have different benefits in the endeavour to understand the person, depending on which of the four domains are currently prominent. In addition, the domains will often appear in specific phases and follow specific trajectories, which can be an argument in favour of a so-called modular structure of the treatment. A prototypical trajectory for many patients with Moderate Personality Disorder could be: (a) establish safety, (b) stop symptom exacerbation, (c) control and regulate emotions and impulses, (d) explore and change more stable maladaptive interpersonal patterns, and (e) integrate and work with more adaptive self-functioning. This would involve a treatment programme divided into different modules that draw on several of the evidence-based psychotherapies. A more behavioural approach is obvious in the first phase, while in later phases you might work more with transference-focused therapy or schema therapy. There are only a few studies that empirically illustrate this approach. An interesting study by Sahin and colleagues (2018) found that a psychodynamic approach had the best effect on Borderline Personality Disorder when symptom severity was low, while there was no difference between psychodynamic therapy and dialectical behaviour therapy when severity was high. One way of making sense of these results is that the psychodynamic treatment provided a better fit or had more to offer to patients with milder disorders struggling less with safety and risk behaviours while being somewhat able to help integrate undesired aspects of the patient's self-identity.

Relationship Between Severity and Treatment Intensity

In many ways it would seem natural that people with the highest severity should also receive the most comprehensive treatment. While this is probably true in many cases, it is not always the case. With the transition to a dimensional system in the coming years, we will know a lot more about this issue. Conceptually and theoretically, the new approach makes it possible to carefully consider various ways severity and treatment levels may interact and test different treatment formats in randomised controlled trials. Treatment of Personality Disorder can have various purposes; for example, stabilisation in an acute crisis phase, long-term support, improving quality of life, and facilitating personality change with the aim of altering aspects of personality functioning and their trait expressions. At the same time, there is great variation in the severity of dysfunction in people with Personality Disorder and their abilities and capabilities. If you consider the many possible interactions among the person's internal and external resources, treatment goals, and treatment formats, it will probably be clear to most clinicians that this is quite complex. On the one hand, people with the most severe Personality Disorders probably also have the highest level of distress and thus potentially the most to gain from long-term and often intensive treatments (Bach & Simonsen, 2021; Goorden et al., 2017). On the other hand, there will also be a group of severely personality disordered patients who function so poorly, both socially and personally, that even very intensive treatments will probably do little more than alleviate acute symptoms. Conversely, people with Mild Personality Disorder will often be able to present themselves in a way that elicits more help (Soeteman et al., 2008). Moreover, they also get more out of the psychotherapeutic programmes, because they already have more resources available than those who are most impaired and disadvantaged (Antonsen et al., 2016). In this way, Personality Disorder poses a significant challenge for service providers when it comes to matching the person to treatment.

The question of adapting treatment to the severity of the Personality Disorder has been the subject of much attention for many years, but only a small handful of studies have sufficient scientific quality to allow us to make clear statements about these issues with a certain degree of certainty. The question of shorter versus longer treatment for patients with Personality Disorder has only been investigated in few studies. One study by McMain and colleagues (2022) found no difference in the effect of 6 versus 12 months of dialectical behaviour therapy. In fact, it seemed that patients in the shorter treatment programme got better faster than those in the longer programme. Along the same lines, a study of short versus long mentalisation-based therapy also showed no difference on any outcomes at 16-months follow up (Juul et al., 2023). Nevertheless, in a secondary analysis of McMain et al.'s study, Traynor et al. (2024) found that more disinhibited patients were specifically doing better in the 6 months treatment programme while those with less disinhibition were doing better in the 12 months treatment programme. Thus, such individual features (i.e., the trait domain of Disinhibition) may be important for clinical management and treatment planning.

Although, on average, there does not seem to be an empirical basis for offering long-term treatment to all individuals with the most severe Personality Disorders, there will probably be a subgroup for whom this is most optimal (Juul et al., 2022). Over the years, various research groups have investigated or described patient characteristics that may help match patients with Personality Disorder to different treatments, often within the framework of a *stepped care* model (Hutsebaut et al., 2020; Simonsen et al., 2017). One of the models that has received the most attention was developed by Lois Choi-Kain et al. (2016). An adapted ICD-11 version of Choi-Kain et al.'s stepped care model is shown in Table 6.2.

Table 6.2   Stepped care model for ICD-11 Personality Disorder severity

Severity	Definition and stage	Interventions	Treatment context
Mild	• Rarely serious risk of harm to self or others • Onset often caused by stressful episodes	• Time-limited group (psycho-dynamic or skills training) or individual psychotherapy • Case management	• Primary care (e.g., private practice psychologist or psychiatrist)
Moderate	• Often risk of harm to self or others • The problems are of a more persistent, serious nature	• Time-limited evidence-based treatment programmes (e.g., DAT, MBT, ST)	• Outpatient psychiatric services

Table 6.2 Continued

Severity	Definition and stage	Interventions	Treatment context
Severe	• Often severe self-harm, serious suicide attempts, and/or risk of violence • Treatment with evidence-based treatments have insufficient effect	• Consider switching from one time-limited therapy to another • Consider adjusting (increasing or decreasing) treatment contact	• Outpatient psychiatric with a higher degree of specialisation and possible inpatient treatment
Chronic persistent disorder	• Risk level corresponding to moderate or severe • Insufficient effect despite repeated treatment attempts with evidence-based treatment	• Supportive care with the aim of increasing quality of life • Generic psychiatric approach takes precedence over specialised evidence-based approach • Probably longer-term contact, but with lower frequency	• Depending on the level of risk, it can be supportive counselling with a private practitioner in primary care or community psychiatric services

Note. DAT = dialectical behaviour therapy; MBT = mentalisation-based therapy; ST = schema therapy.

Currently, many countries offer either inpatient treatment or highly specialised outpatient treatment environments that would be able to adjust and integrate treatments adapted to the individual's current needs (Simonsen et al., 2019). We believe that the implementation of ICD-11 will be an important incentive for the political-administrative management to provide a structural and financial framework recognising the heterogeneous treatment needs of patients with Personality Disorders. Beyond the allocation of clinical resources for different levels of severity, it is certainly also important to consider content and focus of psychotherapy for the different levels. In Table 6.3 and Table 6.4, we propose general and specific guidelines for the therapeutic management of patients with different levels of severity.

Table 6.3   General guidance for therapeutic approach based on severity

Mild	Moderate	Severe
Need less structured and less intensive treatment Little effort is required to maintain the alliance and prevent irreparable ruptures Group therapy is usually sufficient	Need for moderately structured treatment Clinician needs to be more prepared to deal with alliance ruptures, and the risk of dropout is increased	Need highly structured treatment and clear boundary setting Clinician must be very intentional about building alliance, repairing ruptures, and preventing dropout Prioritising suicide and homicide risks, self-harm and violence, and therapy-interfering behaviour

Table 6.4   Suggested treatment strategies based on severity

	Mild	Moderate	Severe
DAT	Focus on interpersonal and other quality of life issues Less comprehensive programmes can be considered (e.g., skills training plus consultation team)	Focus on self-harm and suicidal behaviour, if it occurs Increased focus on other destabilising behaviours, including therapy disruptive behaviour	Primary focus on reducing suicidal and self-harming behaviour, therapy disruptive behaviour, and other severely destabilising behaviours
MBT	Help increase capacity for mentalisation Patients at this level are usually less difficult to reach and are more open to new information due to relatively intact epistemic trust	Help regain mentalisation when lost by rebalancing the poles of mentalization: self–other, affect–cognition, and internal–external	Focus on scaffolding epistemic trust and decreasing epistemic hypervigilance by balancing the patient's need to feel understood and providing a helpful alternative perspective

Table 6.4 Continued

	Mild	Moderate	Severe
ST	Helping the "healthy adult" part of the patient to meet their own emotional needs using empathic confrontation, cognitive behavioural techniques, and experiential work (corrective emotional experiences)	Build the patient's "healthy adult" to fulfil their own emotional needs, while the therapist provides warmth, reassurance, and acceptance to meet the needs that the patient is unable to fulfil, and help the patient integrate different *self-states/ modes*	Compensate for the lack of a "healthy adult" through intensive support and limited reparenting Confront or limit *modes* that are associated with harm to self or others Support integration of dissociated *modes* through experiential work and therapeutic support

Note. DAT = dialectical behaviour therapy; MBT = mentalisation-based therapy; ST = schema therapy.

The Importance of Trait Domains for Treatment

In this book, we have found it appropriate to present severity and trait domains separately, as this seems most helpful in an introduction to the ICD-11 Personality Disorder classification. However, it should be emphasised that this division is somewhat artificial as severity of personality dysfunction is always expressed in certain individual ways ("styles"), which are specified by trait domains. In this section, we will take a closer look at how trait domains can provide a better understanding of the patient and guide us towards a more individualised treatment. While personality functioning can be said to capture how the patients generally "manage" themselves and their relationships, trait domains can be said to further portray the dysfunction that has led to the patient's referral to treatment. As clinicians we should therefore focus our attention on *understanding* the composition of these trait domains in the patient while seeking to *change* the overall level of personality functioning. For example, trait domains can provide a better understanding of individual triggers and stressors that can provoke and amplify the patient's problems (e.g., Negative Affectivity in the form of distrust and emotional lability). From this, we can also consider how we as practitioners can best interact with and establish a good relationship with the patient.

Clinical Considerations for Negative Affectivity

For clinicians, Negative Affectivity is a key domain because it is strongly associated with, for example, emotional crises and suicide risk that are likely to bring the person into contact with the healthcare system. The domain is generally associated with emotional problems and distress that are part of a broader spectrum of mental disorders. Because this domain is highly associated with the act of seeking treatment, virtually all psychotherapeutic models can be interpreted as being orientated towards this domain to a certain degree (Widiger & Trull, 1992). For example, dialectical behaviour therapy targets emotional dysregulation (Linehan & Dexter-Mazza, 2008), Acceptance and commitment therapy focuses on the acceptance of negative affect (Hayes, 2004), and mentalisation-based therapy aims to increase emotional regulation through improved mentalisation skills (Bateman & Fonagy, 2016).

Evidence suggests that the trait domain of Negative Affectivity has a significant impact on Personality Disorders and related problems encountered in general clinical practice. Therefore, Negative Affectivity itself can be considered a *one size fits all* trait domain that also reflects the tendency towards anxiety and depression seen in many consumers of mental health services. However, from a clinical perspective, Negative Affectivity becomes especially useful when seen in combination with other relevant trait domains. Metaphorically, Negative Affectivity can be compared to the alcohol that acts as the base ingredient across many different cocktails. For example, ICD-11 highlights that in combination with Detachment, the domain of Negative Affectivity can cause blame and negativity to be directed towards oneself, whereas in combination with Dissociality, it can involve negativity and blame being directed towards others. Furthermore, ICD-11 recognises that individuals with prominent Negative Affectivity can exhibit low self-esteem in a number of ways depending on context and other dynamics: (a) avoidance of situations that are deemed too difficult, (b) dependence on the advice, guidance, and help of others, (c) envy of others' abilities and indicators of success, and (d) suicidal ideation based on beliefs of being useless in this world. All four variants can even apply to the same person across time and situation, depending on the context, complexity, and severity of the Personality Disorder.

The key message here is that the aforementioned patterns encompass different situational expressions of Negative Affectivity, which point to different implications for treatment. Overall, Negative Affectivity itself can be understood as a transdiagnostic trait domain that applies to all emotional disorders and that, in combination with other domains or factors, can reveal clinically useful information. To further uncover such dynamics of trait domains and severity, it seems worthwhile to investigate and describe the more fine-grained facets of Negative Affectivity. Accordingly, facet-level scales have been developed to describe, for example, emotional lability, negativistic attitudes, low self-esteem, and mistrustfulness (Clark et al., 2021; Oltmanns & Widiger, 2020).

In the context of treatment planning and overall prognosis, a very high or low level of Negative Affectivity will typically be something clinicians should take into account. In many cases, a high level of Negative Affectivity will limit how much you can expect to change the level of distress itself. This does not mean that treatment is ineffective, but simply that it is primarily aimed at, for example, changing how the disorder is expressed or preventing further suffering. Conversely, a very low level of Negative Affectivity can also be problematic in some cases because it can be difficult for the clinician to determine whether this is an expression of a psychological defensiveness or a more genuine lack of emotional vulnerability (Bach, 2020; Bagby et al., 2016).

Clinical Considerations for Detachment

This domain corresponds to the opposite of Extroversion in the classic five-factor model (McCrae, 1991). Individuals who are predominantly characterised by this domain are usually described as shy "loners" that are avoiding intimacy. Seeking treatment may be unusual for people with high levels of Detachment, but some may feel like they are missing out on something crucial in life. Sometimes concerned friends or relatives will arrange for them to get treatment. The key is often to have realistic expectations of the possible change, which involves understanding the patient and, above all, helping them to understand and value themselves (Fischer & Finn, 2008).

One challenge with such patients is that clinicians usually like to be appreciated and gain a sense of progress and personal competence as reflected through the progression of treatment. Patients characterised by Detachment may tend to frustrate the clinician's somewhat "narcissistic" need for appreciation and recognition. Even insightful and psychologically astute observations from the clinician may not elicit any signs of enthusiasm or interest from the patient, and there is a real risk that the clinician's enthusiasm will gradually fade. In the worst-case scenario, this kind of therapeutic narcissism can cause the clinician to show impatience and frustration with the detached person who does not seem to appreciate the therapist's skills and hard work. In such cases, the therapist must be reminded that a good and healthy alliance begins with the therapist primarily focusing on the patient's needs and intentions for coming to treatment. Furthermore, the therapist must also appreciate that the low level of positive affectivity does not mean that the patient is psychologically flat, represses their emotions, or has an intellectually empty existence (Harkness & McNulty, 2006). Sometimes it can be more helpful to change the environment rather than the patient, for example by helping the patient to find their niche (Tyrer, 2002). Mild or moderate Detachment is often seen in people who struggle with low self-esteem and as a result hold themselves back both verbally and non-verbally when they are with other people. Over time, this can have major consequences, both in terms of personality and psychosocial functioning. In many ways, it is natural to think that people with this type of Personality Disorder can learn a lot from individual and/or group therapy, but it is important that the treatment is adapted to problems with lack of initiation and limitations in non-verbal communication (Simonsen et al., 2022).

Clinical Considerations for Dissociality

In many ways, this trait domain corresponds to the opposite of Agreableness in the classic five-factor model (McCrae, 1991). Individuals with prominent Dissociality tend to thwart the therapist's efforts to establish an alliance and cooperation. They can be untrustworthy and will often see other people as the cause of their problems. In some cases, such individuals will be referred to treatment through the legal system. It has been suggested that clinicians considering treating patients with predominant Dissociality should reflect on their own way of confronting unpleasant behaviour without moral condemnation or a tendency to become defensive (Harkness & McNulty, 2006). The therapist should avoid engaging in power struggles or reacting defensively when challenged by the patient's attempts to take control. Some insight into and sensitivity to the patient's worldview can be beneficial.

Treatment goals for Dissociality should be moderated and realistic. Despite resistance and difficulties in establishing an authentic alliance, research suggests that treatment has some effect (Bernstein et al., 2023). One option could be to enter into a collaboration with the patient to uncover whether the dissocial behaviour is worthwhile, that is, whether it may have too many costs for the person. Such an approach would be in concordance with the self-centred aspects of this trait domain, which may be necessary to ensure the right amount of motivation in the patient – because no clinician can make water run uphill.

Clinical Considerations for Disinhibition

This domain essentially corresponds to the opposite of Conscientiousness in the classic five-factor model (McCrae, 1991). Many of the resources associated with Conscientiousness are thus lacking in patients characterised by this trait domain, which manifests as impulsivity, risk taking, lack of persistence, and irresponsibility, among other things. Patients with prominent Disinhibition often enter treatment at the request of concerned family members or friends. The overarching principle of treatment is to help the patient live as constructively as possible with a disinhibited personality style – not to transform the personality into an inhibited, over-controlled, or anankastic version (Harkness & McNulty, 2006).

It has been suggested that Disinhibition in clinical contexts can be equated with Attention Deficit Hyperactivity Disorder (ADHD), which is consistent with research suggesting that facets of Disinhibition, particularly distractibility and impulsivity, are highly related to ADHD (Sellbom et al., 2018; Smith & Samuel, 2017). Treatment will typically involve helping the patient find safer and healthier activities that still fulfil their need for excitement and stimulation.

Clinical Considerations for Anankastia

This domain is associated with a pathologically high level of Conscientiousness according to the five-factor model (McCrae, 1991), which involves perfectionism, emotional and behavioural restrictions, orderliness, and a preoccupation with stubbornly following rules and fulfilling obligations. Again, patients with Anankastia are unlikely to seek treatment because they primarily see the world and other people as the source of disorder, clutter, indiscipline, and moral decay.

An obvious treatment goal in cases where the clinician encounters Anankastia would be to help the patient find more adaptive expressions of their underlying characteristics without expecting these to fundamentally change (Lynch et al., 2015). Individuals with predominant Anankastia usually benefit most from working with specific goals and an active therapist who provides direction, guidance, and sound advice. It can be helpful if the therapist is on time and consistently refers to a structured plan (Bach, 2020). A focus on compassion may make sense to include along the way, when and if self-criticism and strict demands are gradually replaced with greater self-care and acceptance (Gilbert, 2014).

Clinical Interpretation of Combined Trait Domains

Until now, we have focused on trait domains separately, which is a somewhat simplistic and artificial perspective. In clinical practice, it makes the most sense to describe people with more than one prominent trait domain, the combination of which evidently tells us more than the individual elements on their own. This is especially true for patients with moderate to severe Personality Disorders, as complexity usually increases with severity. A more detailed formulation is therefore particularly appropriate for this patient group.

Take, for example, two patients for whom Negative Affectivity is the most prominent trait. One patient is additionally characterised by the trait domain of Dissociality, while the other is additionally characterised by the trait domain of Detachment. The first patient shows externalising anger or over-compensatory grandiosity related to dysregulated emotions and self-esteem. The second patient shows internalising characteristics such as social withdrawal, depressivity, and anxiousness. Clearly, such combinations are informative, and the rest of this chapter describes considerations that have significant implications for treatment planning and goals.

Negative Affectivity and Detachment

This combination essentially means that the person is more likely to experience internalised negative emotions (e.g., anxiousness, depressivity, guilt, inferiority, and pessimism). For example, the person directs blame for failures towards themselves instead of others.

With minimal dysfunction, people with this combination may benefit from the following resources: They are good at predicting potential problems and responding to them independently. They are also very aware of other people's opinions without necessarily having to influence or dominate. Finally, they are self-critical and aware of what they can improve about themselves.

For patients characterised by this combination, treatment should basically help them live a less gloomy and fearful life. There are very few things that can cheer them up, while there are many things that cause them anxiety and suffering. Especially in stressful situations, they tend to become depressed or anxious and long to withdraw from other people. Even under normal circumstances, they tend to find life quite hard and joyless. As a result, they can easily fall into discouragement, despair, and isolation. They let potential problems overshadow opportunities and often suppress their frustrations and anger.

The combination is typically seen in people who were traditionally described as suffering from Avoidant Personality Disorder, that is, people who feel inferior, reserved, and inhibited in relationships and social contact for fear of being criticised or rejected.

In the most severe cases, people with this combination of trait domains may experience confusing, conflicting, illogical, and disturbing feelings and desires. They may be desperate for intimacy (Negative Affectivity) while simultaneously feeling the need to distance themselves from others (Detachment). They may experience high emotional intensity (Negative Affectivity) as well as emotional emptiness, emotional flatness, and anhedonia (Detachment). Such contradictory trait features may also reflect poorly integrated mental models of self and others, which is often seen in severe or extreme impairment of personality functioning.

Negative Affectivity and Dissociality

This combination indicates a propensity to experience externalising negative emotions (e.g., anger, contempt, hostility). They tend to blame others instead of themselves, which can also include holding grudges and having difficulty forgiving others. If they have low self-esteem, it typically manifests as envy of other people's abilities and signs of success.

With minimal dysfunction, people with this combination may be able to utilise the following resources: They are able to respond to conditions or situations that bother them. They are often very direct about their feelings without being blocked by emotional inhibition. And they typically do not suppress their own anger but allow it to be expressed.

People with this combination can benefit from working on their tendency to become enraged over minor annoyances and to hold grudges and resentments for long periods of time. They are deeply self-involved and easily offended, and they often overlook the effects of their anger on others. They may sometimes resort to physical aggression or verbal abuse and at other times be seductive and flattering to gain recognition from others.

In severe cases, individuals with this combination may have an unbalanced and vulnerable self-assessment involving both self-hatred (Negative Affectivity) and an inflated sense of self (Dissociality), sometimes simultaneously in a disintegrated manner or fluctuating between inferiority and self-overestimation. In the most severe cases, they may express their inner pain in violent ways, causing harm to others.

Negative Affectivity and Disinhibition

People with this combination are often at the mercy of their impulses in a negative way. They find it distressing or challenging to resist any urge or desire, and they often lack the self-control and focus to keep their urges in check. As a result, they may act in ways that they know are not in their own best interest and that they will be ashamed of. They may seek short-term pleasures and gratification (e.g., sex, drugs, overeating, and gambling) to regulate or numb negative emotions.

With minimal dysfunction, people with this combination may benefit from being able to act on their feelings and spontaneously do something about their situation (e.g., go for a run instead of just sitting on the couch feeling miserable, or spontaneously invite a friend over).

In the most severe dysfunction, this combination can manifest as self-harming behaviour or careless and potentially dangerous behaviour towards others. There is a risk of substance abuse, eating disorders such as bulimia and binge-eating, and cutting – all destructive alternatives to a spontaneous run in the park.

Negative Affectivity and Anankastia

This combination describes neurotic, rule-bound, perfectionistic, hard-working, indecisive, and doubting individuals who place high demands on themselves. The pattern may involve anankastic attempts to keep difficult emotions under restrictive control, combined with feelings of inadequacy, self-criticism, and shame due to a disproportionate sense of guilt.

Most of the time, this combination will include a propensity and strong need to control their own emotions and actions, causing emotional tension. Such individuals typically have high standards and a perfectionistic drive that does not allow them to fail in the smallest detail (Blatt, 1995). This pattern is often fuelled by low self-esteem and a need to be recognised by others. Because their goals are either unattainable or unrealistic, they are prone to self-criticism, intense feelings of guilt and shame, and burnout. In many cases, their life satisfaction and well-being is compromised by a lack of authenticity.

On the one hand, the combination can characterise the neurotic perfectionist, for whom perfectionism acts as a means to feel adequate, safe, and less vulnerable. On the other hand, perfectionism and orderliness can make a person stressed and vulnerable in a way that perpetuates the pattern in a vicious cycle.

With minimal dysfunction, people with this combination may be able to utilise resources such as the ability to contain their emotions and related impulses to achieve a higher goal. In more severe cases, individuals with this combination can lead to burnout, as well as recurrent and severe depressive episodes and increased suicide risk (Brezo et al., 2006).

Detachment and Disinhibition

This combination may involve that the person is lethargic, unfocused, unmotivated, and without a goal or plan in life. This is a rather rare and paradoxical combination because it encompasses being impulsive and risk taking, combined with being emotionally withdrawn, emotionally flat, and socially withdrawn. It can be a withdrawal from the distractions and chores often associated with social relationships. Individuals with this combination may also have difficulty making and following through on plans, including social activities, which perpetuates their status as loners. In general, impulse control issues can lead to defeat and shame, which ultimately perpetuates and reinforces their withdrawal and isolation. Individuals with this pattern can thus be "lone wolves" who mostly see other people as distractions and do not want to take initiative, engage in social obligations, or be responsible for the well-being of others. They can easily forget appointments and be sluggish in their infrequent attempts to maintain any social relationships. Furthermore, when in social and interpersonal situations, they may feel so distracted and indifferent that they prefer not to be interpersonally involved. Their hedonic capacity can be significantly limited. At times, they may be emotionally flat, mute or closed off, and unconcerned about risks, which may create danger for themselves or others.

In the most critical cases, clinicians should be aware that this combination may indicate early signs of Schizophrenia in the form of cognitive disturbances, motivational problems, and distractibility, along with social isolation, withdrawal, and anhedonia (all so-called negative symptoms). This is particularly noteworthy when there is a severe degree of compromised reality testing as an aspect of cognitive manifestations (Ohi et al., 2016). In other cases, this pattern may also characterise aspects of Attention Deficit Disorder (ADD), ADHD, and mentally absent-minded and daydreaming individuals, who often tend to withdraw or "zone out" from the outside world.

Dissociality and Detachment

This combination can include callous and unemotional features both due to emotional detachment as well as emotional coldness, which in mild to moderate cases can characterise a *lone ranger*. Such individuals are indifferent to the opinions and well-being of other people and may view everyone as a potential enemy if they come in their way. They rarely settle down or form close bonds and can easily move from one place to another. However, their withdrawn and cynical style can cause suffering to those around them. These individuals are often cunning, distant, and keep to themselves, while their loved ones (if they have any) can feel emotionally deprived and hurt with no chance of relational repair or comfort.

People with this combination of traits will typically favour respect over friendship and closeness. They tend to value their privacy so, when interacting with them, it is wise to give them the space they need.

With minimal dysfunction, individuals with this combination may be able to capitalise on resources such as an ability to compete and stay focused on the goal while eliminating potential obstacles, including their own emotional distractions. In the most severe cases, individuals with this combination may view interpersonal relationships purely as a tool for personal gain, which is rarely reciprocated. Furthermore, they may be unable to appreciate the experiences, perspectives, and motivations of others. If this combination is further accompanied by a marked absence of Negative Affectivity (stress immunity and fearlessness), a form of psychopathy may be present (Anderson et al., 2014). Due to their emotional and interpersonal detachment they may not exhibit much activity but, when they act, it might be in cold blood without being under the influence of emotions.

Dissociality and Disinhibition

This combination can involve both being indifferent to other people (e.g., cynicism and lack of empathy) and disregard for the safety of others (e.g., reckless behaviour). Individuals characterised by these traits are typically more concerned with their own gratification than the well-being of others. They are risk seeking, spontaneous, and not only inconsiderate of other people, but basically indifferent to them. They also tend to be unable of sustained effort (i.e., weak willed) and often have some undesirable habits (e.g., drugs, gambling, impulse buying, casual sex) that are difficult for them to stop. Such people are easily bored, procrastinate, seek out stimulation, behave impulsively and irresponsibly, and live a parasitic lifestyle without planning, while opportunistically exploiting other people's patience, trust, and ability to maintain housing and jobs, which they can then prey on until something better comes along. If this combination is further supplemented with Negative Affectivity, the clinicians should pay attention to the risk of unpredictable, explosive, and uncalculated aggression.

Dissociality and Anankastia

This combination characterises people who are first and foremost concerned with their own needs and are effective in pursuing their own goals and fighting for their own interests. They are know-it-all, ruthless, bureaucratic, and uncompromising. They are often perceived by others as narcissists or control freaks who make unreasonably high demands. They may succeed in politics, administration, or business because of their determined persistence. The pattern can also describe a bureaucratic and entitled form of Anankastia, which characterises those in positions of authority in organisations and boards who act pettily and vindictively towards others. Such individuals often manage to suppress, sublimate, and transform their Dissociality to detect and punish mistakes and rule breaking in the public interest, for example, in roles such as supervisors, police officers, activists, and judges who fulfil their own needs for power and control in their work rather than serving the community in a more pragmatic and inclusive manner. Finally, people with this combination of traits may be so proud and conscious of their own perfection and efficient way of doing things that they feel superior to most other people.

Anankastia and Detachment

This combination indicates a pervasive restriction or "rigidity" that manifests itself both interpersonally and emotionally. Individuals characterised by this combination are thus careful to the point of being "stingy" with emotional expression or social contact because they are trying to protect themselves from losing face or to safeguard against the unwanted intrusion of others into their psychological space. They can sometimes be puritanical and frugal kinds of people who dogmatically seek to control and counteract their own repulsive impulses and fantasies. The pattern can also involve being overly goal orientated and preoccupied with productivity and perfection to the exclusion of unnecessary interpersonal relationships, pleasures, and joys. Such individuals may be so focused on the task at hand and their own flawless way of doing it that they only ask others for help when it is absolutely necessary, in which case it must be done in a very specific way. Furthermore, they typically view emotions as irrational artefacts that do not really serve any purpose in life. In severe cases, the fear of letting others get close can be said to be rooted in paranoid distrust rather than self-doubt.

With minimal dysfunction, people with this combination can often be good "methodical" workers, concentrating on the task at hand and working at a steady pace until the work is completed. They cannot rush, but they can be counted on to complete their tasks. Thus, they are good at staying organised and meticulously getting things done correctly despite (or because of) not relying on the assistance or company of others. Such trait combination can be advantageous in situations where a high degree of safety, perfection, reliability, and independence is required (e.g., criminal investigators, aircraft mechanics).

Anankastia and Disinhibition

This combination may seem contradictory and paradoxical because Anankastia is commonly considered the opposite pole to Disinhibition, based on a continuum between Anankastia and Disinhibition with dysfunction at both ends. However, research suggests that Anankastia is more than just extremely high Conscientiousness or extremely low Disinhibition (Bach, Kerber et al., 2020; Saulsman & Page, 2004). Perfectionistic individuals with low levels of Disinhibition may have enough flexibility to direct their attention to the task at hand, whereas individuals with high levels of Anankastia may strive for perfection and order in a way that actually compromises their ability to complete the task at hand while also generating stress, disorder, and chaotic thinking. For example, the excessive focus on detail, productivity, order, and constantly having to "check" that everything is in order (Anankastia) can also produce quite a lot of distractibility (Disinhibition). Therefore, from a clinical perspective, it is not surprising that people with challenges related to Anankastia can also be burdened by certain characteristics of Disinhibition (Villemarette-Pittman et al., 2004).

Another dynamic may be that Disinhibition sometimes characterises individuals with ADD/ADHD (Smith & Samuel, 2017). These individuals may have developed enduring anankastic or compulsive patterns to compensate for the chaos that often characterises Disinhibition. Furthermore, anankastic rigidity and perseveration can sometimes manifest in individuals with ADD/ADHD in the form of stubbornness and "hyperfocus" when, for example, the ability to switch from one task to another is impaired (Barkley, 2018).

In more severe cases of personality dysfunction, this combination of traits may reflect that the person is disturbed by conflicting and incoherent internal demands. In some situations, or conditions, such individuals may have unreasonably high and restrictive personal standards (Anankastia), while at other times or in other conditions they may have irresponsibly low and care-less personal standards (Disinhibition).

The Misery Triad: Negative Affectivity, Disinhibition, and Detachment

Clinicians need to pay special attention to this combination, which indicates a general misery that significantly affects the person's well-being, prognosis, and course of treatment (Miller, 1991). The prevalence of Negative Affectivity means that the person feels anxious, depressed, and worthless. Detachment involves the person not sharing their experience with anyone or seeking help to alleviate the disorder. Finally, Disinhibition means that the person is unable to do anything constructive about the problems or the disorder, such as organising their daily life and setting goals to feel better. Together, this triad of trait domains creates a vicious circle that can easily spiral out of control and be extremely difficult to escape. If the patient already suffers from self-hatred and suicidal thoughts as an aspect of Negative Affectivity, it is especially important to be aware that it can be very difficult for the individual to move on and distance themselves from these thoughts. In addition, there may be an increased risk of self-medication in the form of substance abuse or attempts to numb negative emotions through gambling or other addictions, which can also be quite challenging for such individuals to recover from.

References

Allen, A., & Links, P. S. (2012). Aggression in borderline personality disorder: Evidence for increased risk and clinical predictors. *Current Psychiatry Reports, 14*(1), 62–69. https://doi.org/10.1007/s11920-011-0244-9

Allport, G. W. (1937). *Personality: A psychological interpretation*. University of Michigan.

Alnæs, R., & Torgersen, S. (1988). The relationship between DSM-III symptom disorders (Axis I) and personality disorders (Axis II) in an outpatient population. *Acta Psychiatrica Scandinavica, 78*(4), 485–492. https://doi.org/10.1111/j.1600-0447.1988.tb06371.x

American Psychiatric Association, DSM-5 Task Force. (2013). *Diagnostic and statistical manual of mental disorders: DSM-5* (5th ed.). American Psychiatric Publishing.

Anderson, J. L., Sellbom, M., Wygant, D. B., Salekin, R. T., & Krueger, R. F. (2014). Examining the associations between DSM-5 section III antisocial personality disorder traits and psychopathy in community and university samples. *Journal of Personality Disorders, 28*(5), 675–697. https://doi.org/10.1521/pedi_2014_28_134

Antonsen, B. T., Johansen, M. S., Rø, F. G., Kvarstein, E. H., & Wilberg, T. (2016). Is reflective functioning associated with clinical symptoms and long-term course in patients with personality disorders? *Comprehensive Psychiatry, 64*, 46–58. https://doi.org/10.1016/j.comppsych.2015.05.016

Arnold, S. R., Higgins, J. M., Weise, J., Desai, A., Pellicano, E., & Trollor, J. N. (2023). Confirming the nature of autistic burnout. *Autism, 27*(7), 1906–1918. https://doi.org/10.1177/13623613221147410

Aydın-Seyrek, T., Gandur, T., Turgut, N., Kunt, D. A., & Dereboy, F. (2024). Reliability of the ICD-11 personality disorder severity ratings and diagnosis. *Personality and Mental Health*. Advance online publication. https://doi.org/10.1002/pmh.1629

Bach, B. (2020). Simplicity and dynamics of the ICD-11 trait qualifiers in relation to treatment. In K. L. Gratz & C. Lejuez (Eds.), *The Cambridge Handbook of Personality Disorders* (pp. 475–476). Cambridge University Press. https://doi.org/10.1017/9781108333931.082

Bach, B., Brown, T. A., Mulder, R. T., Newton-Howes, G., Simonsen, E., & Sellbom, M. (2021). Development and initial evaluation of the ICD-11 personality disorder severity scale: PDS-ICD-11. *Personality and Mental Health, 15*(3), 223–236. https://doi.org/10.1002/pmh.1510

Bach, B., Christensen, S., Kongerslev, M. T., Sellbom, M., & Simonsen, E. (2020). Structure of clinician-reported ICD-11 personality disorder trait qualifiers. *Psychological Assessment, 32*(1), 50–59. https://doi.org/10.1037/pas0000747

Bach, B., & First, M. B. (2018). Application of the ICD-11 classification of personality disorders. *BMC Psychiatry, 18*(1), Article 351.

Bach, B., & Hutsebaut, J. (2018). Level of Personality Functioning Scale – brief form 2.0: Utility in capturing personality problems in psychiatric outpatients and incarcerated addicts. *Journal of Personality Assessment, 100*(6), 660–670.

Bach, B., Kerber, A., Aluja, A., Bastiaens, T., Keeley, J. W., Claes, L., Fossati, A., Gutierrez, F., Oliveira, S. E. S., Pires, R., Riegel, K. D., Rolland, J.-P., Roskam, I., Sellbom, M., Somma, A., Spanemberg, L., Strus, W., Thimm, J. C., Wright, A. G. C., ... Zimmermann, J. (2020). International assessment of DSM-5 and ICD-11 personality disorder traits: Toward a common nosology in DSM-5.1. *Psychopathology, 53*(3–4), 179–188.

Bach, B., Kramer, U., Doering, S., di Giacomo, E., Hutsebaut, J., Kaera, A., De Panfilis, C., Schmahl, C., Swales, M., Taubner, S., & Renneberg, B. (2022). The ICD-11 classification of personality disorders: A European perspective on challenges and opportunities. *Borderline Personality Disorder and Emotion Dysregulation, 9*(1), 12. https://doi.org/10.1186/s40479-022-00182-0

Bach, B., & Mulder, R. (2022). Clinical implications of ICD-11 for diagnosing and treating personality disorders. *Current Psychiatry Reports, 24*(10), 553–563. https://doi.org/10.1007/s11920-022-01364-x

Bach, B., & Presnall-Shvorin, J. (2020). Using DSM-5 and ICD-11 personality traits in clinical treatment. In C. W. Lejuez & K. L. Gratz (Eds.), *The Cambridge Handbook of Personality Disorders* (pp. 450–467). Cambridge University Press. https://doi.org/10.1017/9781108333931.079

Bach, B., Sellbom, M., Kongerslev, M. T., Simonsen, E., Krueger, R. F., & Mulder, R. T. (2017). Deriving ICD-11 personality disorder domains from DSM-5 traits: Initial attempt to harmonize two diagnostic systems. *Acta Psychiatrica Scandinavica, 136*(1), 108–117. https://doi.org/10.1111/acps.12748

Bach, B., Sellbom, M., Skjernov, M., & Simonsen, E. (2018). ICD-11 and DSM-5 personality trait domains capture categorical personality disorders: Finding a common ground. *Australian & New Zealand Journal of Psychiatry, 52*(5), 425–434. https://doi.org/10.1177/0004867417727867

Bach, B., & Sellbom, M. (2025). *Diagnostic Interview for Personality Pathology in ICD-11 (DIPP-11)*. Hogrefe.

Bach, B., Simonsen, E., Kongerslev, M. T., Bo, S., Hastrup, L. H., Simonsen, S., & Sellbom, M. (2023). ICD-11 personality disorder features in the Danish general population: Cutoffs and prevalence rates for severity levels. *Psychiatry Research, 328*, 115484. https://doi.org/10.1016/j.psychres.2023.115484

Bach, B., & Simonsen, S. (2021). How does level of personality functioning inform clinical management and treatment? Implications for ICD-11 classification of personality disorder severity. *Current Opinion in Psychiatry, 34*(1), 54–63. https://doi.org/10.1097/YCO.0000000000000658

Bach, B., & Tracy, M. (2022). Clinical utility of the alternative model of personality disorders: A 10th year anniversary review. *Personality Disorders: Theory, Research, and Treatment, 13*(4), 369–379. https://doi.org/10.1037/per0000527

Bach, B., & Vestergaard, M. (2023). Differential diagnosis of ICD-11 personality disorder and autism spectrum disorder in adolescents. *Children, 10*(6), 992. https://doi.org/10.3390/children10060992

Bagby, R. M., Gralnick, T. M., Al-Dajani, N., & Uliaszek, A. A. (2016). The role of the five-factor model in personality assessment and treatment planning. *Clinical Psychology: Science and Practice, 23*(4), 365–381. https://doi.org/10.1111/cpsp.12175

Barkley, R. A. (2018). *Attention-deficit hyperactivity disorder: A handbook for diagnosis and treatment* (4th ed.). Guilford Press.

Bateman, A. W. (2011). Throwing the baby out with the bathwater? *Personality and Mental Health, 5*(4), 274–280. https://doi.org/10.1002/pmh.184

Bateman, A. W., & Fonagy, P. (2016). *Mentalization based treatment for personality disorders: A practical guide*. Oxford University Press. https://doi.org/10.1093/med:psych/9780199680375.001.0001

Bateman, A. W., Gunderson, J. G., & Mulder, R. T. (2015). Treatment of personality disorder. *The Lancet, 385*(9969), 735–743.

Baumeister, R. F., & Leary, M. R. (1995). The need to belong: Desire for interpersonal attachments as a fundamental human motivation. *Psychological Bulletin, 117*(3), 497–529. https://doi.org/10.1037/0033-2909.117.3.497

Beatson, J. A., Broadbear, J. H., Duncan, C., Bourton, D., & Rao, S. (2019). Avoiding misdiagnosis when auditory verbal hallucinations are present in borderline personality disorder. *Journal of Nervous and Mental Disease, 207*(12), 1048–1055. https://doi.org/10.1097/NMD.0000000000001073

Beckwith, H., Moran, P. F., & Reilly, J. (2014). Personality disorder prevalence in psychiatric outpatients: A systematic literature review. *Personality and Mental Health, 8*(2), 91–101. https://doi.org/10.1002/pmh.1252

Bender, D. S. (2019). The P-factor and what it means to be human: Commentary on criterion A of the AMPD in HiTOP. *Journal of Personality Assessment, 101*(4), 356–359. https://doi.org/10.1080/00223891.2018.1492928

Bender, D. S. (2005). The therapeutic alliance in the treatment of personality disorders. *Journal of Psychiatric Practice, 11*(2), 73–87. https://doi.org/10.1097/00131746-200503000-00002

Bernstein, D. P., Iscan, C., Maser, J., Boards of Directors of the Association for Research in Personality Disorders, & International Society for the Study of Personality Disorders (2007). Opinions of personality disorder experts regarding the DSM-IV personality disorders classification system. *Journal of Personality Disorders, 21*(5), 536–551.

Bernstein, D. P., Keulen-de Vos, M., Clercx, M., de Vogel, V., Kersten, G. C. M., Lancel, M., Jonkers, P. P., Bogaerts, S., Slaats, M., Broers, N. J., Deenen, T. A. M., & Arntz, A. (2023). Schema therapy for violent PD offenders: A randomized clinical trial. *Psychological Medicine, 53*(1), 88–102.

Blatt, S. J. (1995). The destructiveness of perfectionism: Implications for the treatment of depression. *American Psychologist, 50*(12), 1003–1020. https://doi.org/10.1037/0003-066X.50.12.1003

Blay, M., Cham, M.-A., Duarte, M., & Ronningstam, E. (2024). Association between pathological narcissism and emotion dysregulation: A systematic review. *Psychopathology, 57*(4), 297–317. https://doi.org/10.1159/000538546

Blüml, V., & Doering, S. (2021). ICD-11 personality disorders: A psychodynamic perspective on personality functioning. *Frontiers in Psychiatry, 12*(April), 1–8. https://doi.org/10.3389/fpsyt.2021.654026

Bohus, M., Stoffers-Winterling, J., Sharp, C., Krause-Utz, A., Schmahl, C., & Lieb, K. (2021). Borderline personality disorder. *The Lancet, 398*(10310), 1528–1540. https://doi.org/10.1016/S0140-6736(21)00476-1

Bornstein, R. F., Becker-Matero, N., Winarick, D. J., & Reichman, A. L. (2010). Interpersonal dependency in borderline personality disorder: Clinical context and empirical evidence. *Journal of Personality Disorders, 24*(1), 109–127. https://doi.org/10.1521/pedi.2010.24.1.109

Bradley, L., Shaw, R., Baron-Cohen, S., & Cassidy, S. (2021). Autistic adults' experiences of camouflaging and its perceived impact on mental health. *Autism in Adulthood, 3*(4), 320–329. https://doi.org/10.1089/aut.2020.0071

Brezo, J., Paris, J., & Turecki, G. (2006). Personality traits as correlates of suicidal ideation, suicide attempts, and suicide completions: A systematic review. *Acta Psychiatrica Scandinavica, 113*(3), 180–206. https://doi.org/10.1111/j.1600-0447.2005.00702.x

Brown, T. A., Sellbom, M., Bach, B., & Newton-Howes, G. (2023). New Zealand (Aotearoa) clinicians' perspectives on the utility of the ICD-11 personality disorder diagnosis. *Personality and Mental Health, 17*(3), 282–291. https://doi.org/10.1002/pmh.1582

Caligor, E., Kernberg, O. F., Clarkin, J. F., & Yeomans, F. E. (2018). *Psychodynamic therapy for personality pathology: Treating self and interpersonal functioning.* American Psychiatric Association Publishing. https://doi.org/10.1176/appi.books.9781615373529

Carnovale, M., Carlson, E. N., Quilty, L. C., & Bagby, R. M. (2019). Discrepancies in self- and informant-reports of personality pathology: Examining the DSM–5 Section III trait model. *Personality Disorders: Theory, Research, and Treatment, 10*(5), 456–467. https://doi.org/10.1037/per0000342

Carpenter, R. W., & Trull, T. J. (2013). Components of emotion dysregulation in borderline personality disorder: A review. *Current Psychiatry Reports, 15*(1), 335. https://doi.org/10.1007/s11920-012-0335-2

Carroll, A., Walvisch, J., & Marsh, T. (2022). Personality disorders and forensic assessments: The benefits of ICD-11. *Medicine, Science and the Law, 62*(4), 285–291. https://doi.org/10.1177/00258024221094188

Chanen, A. M., & McCutcheon, L. K. (2008). Personality disorder in adolescence: The diagnosis that dare not speak its name. *Personality and Mental Health, 2*(1), 35–41. https://doi.org/10.1002/pmh.28

Chanen, A. M., Sharp, C., Nicol, K., & Kaess, M. (2022). Early intervention for personality disorder. *FOCUS, 20*(4), 402–408. https://doi.org/10.1176/appi.focus.20220062

Choi-Kain, L. W., Albert, E. B., & Gunderson, J. G. (2016). Evidence-based treatments for borderline personality disorder: Implementation, integration, and stepped care. *Harvard Review of Psychiatry, 24*(5), 342–356. https://doi.org/10.1097/HRP.0000000000000113

Clark, L. A. (2007). Assessment and diagnosis of personality disorder: Perennial issues and an emerging reconceptualization. *Annual Review of Psychology, 58*, 227–257. https://doi.org/10.1146/annurev.psych.57.102904.190200

Clark, L. A., Corona-Espinosa, A., Khoo, S., Kotelnikova, Y., Levin-Aspenson, H. F., Serapio-García, G., & Watson, D. (2021). Preliminary scales for ICD-11 personality disorder: Self and interpersonal dysfunction plus five personality disorder trait domains. *Frontiers in Psychology, 12*. https://doi.org/10.3389/fpsyg.2021.668724

Clark, L. A., Nuzum, H., & Ro, E. (2018). Manifestations of personality impairment severity: Comorbidity, course/prognosis, psychosocial dysfunction, and "borderline" personality features. *Current Opinion in Psychology, 21*, 117–121. https://doi.org/10.1016/j.copsyc.2017.12.004

Clarkin, J. F., Cain, N., & Livesley, W. J. (2015). An integrated approach to treatment of patients with personality disorders. *Journal of Psychotherapy Integration, 25*(1), 3–12. https://doi.org/10.1037/a0038766

Cook, J., Hull, L., Crane, L., & Mandy, W. (2021). Camouflaging in autism: A systematic review. *Clinical Psychology Review, 89*, 102080. https://doi.org/10.1016/j.cpr.2021.102080

Crawford, M. J., Koldobsky, N., Mulder, R. T., & Tyrer, P. (2011). Classifying personality disorder according to severity. *Journal of Personality Disorders, 25*(3), 321–330. https://doi.org/10.1521/pedi.2011.25.3.321

D'Agostino, A., Rossi Monti, M., & Starcevic, V. (2019). Psychotic symptoms in borderline personality disorder. *Current Opinion in Psychiatry, 32*(1), 22–26. https://doi.org/10.1097/YCO.0000000000000462

D'Aurizio, G., Di Stefano, R., Socci, V., Rossi, A., Barlattani, T., Pacitti, F., & Rossi, R. (2023). The role of emotional instability in borderline personality disorder: A systematic review. *Annals of General Psychiatry, 22*(1), 9. https://doi.org/10.1186/s12991-023-00439-0

Darling Rasmussen, P. (2023). "I was never broken – I just don't fit in this world": A case report series of misdiagnosed women with higher functioning ASD. *Nordic Journal of Psychiatry, 77*(4), 352–359. https://doi.org/10.1080/08039488.2022.2112973

Davidson, K. (2011). Changing the classification of personality disorders: An ICD-11 proposal that goes too far? *Personality and Mental Health, 5*(4), 243–245. https://doi.org/10.1002/pmh.180

Day, N. J. S., Green, A., Denmeade, G., Bach, B., & Grenyer, B. F. S. (2024). Narcissistic personality disorder in the ICD-11: Severity and trait profiles of grandiosity and vulnerability. *Journal of Clinical Psychology, 80*(8), 1917–1936. https://doi.org/10.1002/jclp.23701

Ekselius, L., Lindström, E., Knorring, L., Bodlund, O., & Kullgren, G. (1993). Personality disorders in DSM-III-R as categorical or dimensional. *Acta Psychiatrica Scandinavica, 88*(3), 183–187. https://doi.org/10.1111/j.1600-0447.1993.tb03436.x

Evans, S. C., Reed, G. M., Roberts, M. C., Esparza, P., Watts, A. D., Correia, J. M., Ritchie, P., Maj, M., & Saxena, S. (2013). Psychologists' perspectives on the diagnostic classification of mental disorders: Results from the WHO-IUPsyS Global Survey. *International Journal of Psychology, 48*(3), 177–193. https://doi.org/10.1080/00207594.2013.804189

Fang, S., Ouyang, Z., Zhang, P., He, J., Fan, L., Luo, X., Zhang, J., Xiong, Y., Luo, F., Wang, X., Yao, S., & Wang, X. (2021). Personality Inventory for DSM-5 in China: Evaluation of DSM-5 and ICD-11 trait structure and continuity with personality disorder types. *Frontiers in Psychiatry*, 12. https://doi.org/10.3389/fpsyt.2021.635214

Fassbinder, E., & Arntz, A. (2018). Schema therapy with emotionally inhibited and fearful patients. *Journal of Contemporary Psychotherapy, 49*(1), 7–14. https://doi.org/10.1007/s10879-018-9396-9

Fazel, S., & Danesh, J. (2002). Serious mental disorder in 23 000 prisoners: A systematic review of 62 surveys. *The Lancet, 359*(9306), 545–550.

Felding, S. U., Mikkelsen, L. B., & Bach, B. (2021). Complex PTSD and personality disorder in ICD-11: When to assign one or two diagnoses? *Australasian Psychiatry, 29*(6), 590–594. https://doi.org/10.1177/10398562211014212

First, M. B., Skodol, A. E., Bender, D. S., & Oldham, J. M. (2018). *Structured clinical interview for the DSM-5 alternative model for personality disorders (SCID-AMPD)*. American Psychiatric Association Publishing.

Fischer, C. T., & Finn, S. E. (2008). Developing the life meaning of psychological test data: Collaborative and therapeutic approaches. In R. P. Archer & S. R. Smith (Eds.), *Personality Assessment* (pp. 379–404). Routledge.

Fjermestad-Noll, J., Ronningstam, E., Bach, B., Rosenbaum, B., & Simonsen, E. (2020). Perfectionism, shame, and aggression in depressive patients with narcissistic personality disorder. *Journal of Personality Disorders, 34*, 25–41. https://doi.org/10.1521/pedi.2020.34.supp.25

Folmo, E. J., Stänicke, E., Johansen, M. S., Pedersen, G., & Kvarstein, E. H. (2021). Development of therapeutic alliance in mentalization-based treatment: Goals, bonds, and tasks in a specialized treatment for borderline personality disorder. *Psychotherapy Research, 31*(5), 604–618. https://doi.org/10.1080/10503307.2020.1831097

Fombonne, E. (2020). Camouflage and autism. *Journal of Child Psychology and Psychiatry, 61*(7), 735–738. https://doi.org/10.1111/jcpp.13296

Fonagy, P., & Allison, E. (2016). Psychic reality and the nature of consciousness. *The International Journal of Psychoanalysis, 97*(1), 5–24.

Fonagy, P., & Target, M. (2003). *Psychoanalytic theories: Perspectives from developmental psychopathology*. Whurr.

Frances, A. (1980). The DSM-III personality disorders section: A commentary. *American Journal of Psychiatry, 137*(9), 1050–1054. https://doi.org/10.1176/ajp.137.9.1050

Freeman, A. M., & Beck, A. T. (1990). *Cognitive therapy of personality disorders* (1st ed.). Guilford Press.

Frederiksen, C., Solbakken, O. A., Licht, R. W., Jørgensen, C. R., Rodrigo-Domingo, M., & Kjaersdam Telléus, G. (2021). Emotional dysfunction in avoidant personality disorder and borderline personality disorder: A cross-sectional comparative study. *Scandinavian Journal of Psychology, 62*(6), 878–886. https://doi.org/10.1111/sjop.12771

Gamache, D., Savard, C., Leclerc, P., Payant, M., Berthelot, N., Côté, A., Faucher, J., Lampron, M., Lemieux, R., Mayrand, K., Nolin, M., & Tremblay, M. (2021). A proposed classification of ICD-11 severity degrees of personality pathology using the self and interpersonal functioning scale. *Frontiers in Psychiatry, 12*. https://doi.org/10.3389/fpsyt.2021.628057

García, L. F., Aluja, A., Urieta, P., & Gutiérrez, F. (2022). High convergent validity among the five-factor model, PID-5-SF, and PiCD. *Personality Disorders: Theory, Research, and Treatment, 13*(2), 119–132. https://doi.org/10.1037/per0000486

Gilbert, P. (2014). The origins and nature of compassion focused therapy. *British Journal of Clinical Psychology, 53*(1), 6–41. https://doi.org/10.1111/bjc.12043

Goodwin, R. D., Cox, B. J., & Clara, I. (2006). Neuroticism and physical disorders among adults in the community: Results from the national comorbidity survey. *Journal of Behavioral Medicine, 29*(3), 229–238. https://doi.org/10.1007/s10865-006-9048-5

Goorden, M., Willemsen, E. M. C., Bouwmans-Frijters, C. A. M., Busschbach, J. J. V, Noomx, M. J., van der Feltz-Cornelis, C. M., Uyl-de Groot, C. A., & Hakkaart-van Roijen, L. (2017). Developing a decision tool to identify patients with personality disorders in need of highly specialized care. *BMC Psychiatry, 17*(1), 317. https://doi.org/10.1037/t64878-000

Goth, K., Birkhölzer, M., & Schmeck, K. (2018). Assessment of personality functioning in adolescents with the LoPF-Q 12–18 self-report questionnaire. *Journal of Personality Assessment, 100*(6), 680–690. https://doi.org/10.1080/00223891.2018.1489258

Gutiérrez, F., Aluja, A., Rodríguez, C., Gárriz, M., Peri, J. M., Gallart, S., Calvo, N., Ferrer, M., Gutiérrez-Zotes, A., Soler, J., Pascual, J. C., Gutiérrez-Zotes, A., Soler, J., & Pascual, J. C. (2022). Severity in the ICD-11 personality disorder model: Evaluation in a Spanish mixed sample. *Frontiers in Psychiatry, 13*.

Gutiérrez, F., Aluja, A., Ruiz Rodríguez, J., Peri, J. M., Gárriz, M., Garcia, L. F., Sorrel, M. A., Sureda, B., Vall, G., Ferrer, M., & Calvo, N. (2023). Borderline, where are you? A psychometric approach to the personality domains in the International Classification of Diseases, 11th Revision (ICD-11). *Personality Disorders: Theory, Research, and Treatment, 14*(3), 355–359.

Hansen, S. J., Christensen, S., Kongerslev, M. T., First, M. B., Widiger, T. A., Simonsen, E., & Bach, B. (2019). Mental health professionals' perceived clinical utility of the ICD-10 vs. ICD-11 classification of personality disorders. *Personality and Mental Health, 13*(2), 84–95.

Harkness, A. R., & McNulty, J. L. (2006). An overview of personality: The MMPI-2 personality psychopathology five (PSY-5) scales. In J. N. Butcher (Ed.), *MMPI-2: A practitioner's guide* (pp. 73–97). American Psychological Association.

Hayes, S. (2004). Acceptance and commitment therapy and the new behavior therapies: Mindfulness, acceptance, and relationship. Mindfulness and Acceptance. *Expanding the Cognitive-Behavioral Tradition, 35*(4), 639–665.

Hemmati, A., Rahmani, F., & Bach, B. (2021). The ICD-11 personality disorder trait model fits the Kurdish population better than the DSM-5 trait model. *Frontiers in Psychiatry, 12*. https://doi.org/10.3389/fpsyt.2021.635813

Herpertz, S. C., Huprich, S. K., Bohus, M., Chanen, A. M., Goodman, M., Mehlum, L., Moran, P., Newton-Howes, G., Scott, L., & Sharp, C. (2017). The challenge of transforming the diagnostic system of personality disorders. *Journal of Personality Disorders, 31*(5), 577–589. https://doi.org/10.1521/pedi_2017_31_338

Hopwood, C. J. (2018). A framework for treating DSM-5 alternative model for personality disorder features. *Personality and Mental Health, 12*(2), 107–125. https://doi.org/10.1002/pmh.1414

Hopwood, C. J., Bagby, R. M., Gralnick, T., Ro, E., Ruggero, C., Mullins-Sweatt, S., Kotov, R., Bach, B., Cicero, D. C., Krueger, R. F., Patrick, C. J., Chmielewski, M., DeYoung, C. G., Docherty, A. R., Eaton, N. R., Forbush, K. T., Ivanova, M. Y., Latzman, R. D., Pincus, A. L., ... Zimmermann, J. (2020). Integrating psychotherapy with the hierarchical taxonomy of psychopathology (HiTOP). *Journal of Psychotherapy Integration, 30*(4), 477–497.

Hopwood, C. J., Donnellan, M. B., Blonigen, D. M., Krueger, R. F., McGue, M., Iacono, W. G., & Burt, S. A. (2011). Genetic and environmental influences on personality trait stability and growth during the transition to adulthood: A three-wave longitudinal study. *Journal of Personality and Social Psychology, 100*(3), 545–556. https://doi.org/10.1037/e566572011-001

Hopwood, C. J., Malone, J. C., Ansell, E. B., Sanislow, C. A., Grilo, C. M., McGlashan, T. H., Pinto, A., Markowitz, J. C., Shea, M. T., Skodol, A. E., Gunderson, J. G., Zanarini, M. C., & Morey, L. C. (2011). Personality assessment in DSM-5: empirical support for rating severity, style, and traits. *Journal of Personality Disorders, 25*(3), 305–320.

Hopwood, C. J., & Sellbom, M. (2013). Implications of DSM-5 personality traits for forensic psychology. *Psychological Injury and Law, 6*(4), 314–323. https://doi.org/10.1007/s12207-013-9176-5

Horney, K. (2013). *Our inner conflicts: A constructive theory of neurosis* (Vol. 17). Routledge.

Hörz-Sagstetter, S., Ohse, L., & Kampe, L. (2021). Three dimensional approaches to personality disorders: A review on personality functioning, personality structure, and personality organization. *Current Psychiatry Reports, 23*(7), 45. https://doi.org/10.1007/s11920-021-01250-y

Hualparuca-Olivera, L., Calle-Arancibia, M., Caycho-Rodríguez, T., & Bach, B. (2024). Self-reported ICD-11 personality disorder severity in Peruvian adolescents: Structure, validity, and tentative cutoffs. *Journal of Personality Disorders, 38*(4), 401–413. https://doi.org/10.1521/pedi.2024.38.4.401

Hualparuca-Olivera, L., Caycho-Rodríguez, T., Torales, J., Ramos-Vera, C., Ramos-Campos, D., Córdova-Gónzales, L., & Bach, B. (2024). Internal consistency of measures for ICD-11 personality disorder severity and traits: A systematic review and meta-analysis.

Personality and Mental Health. Advance online publication. https://doi.org/10.1002/pmh.1631

Huprich, S. K. (2013). New directions for an old construct: Depressive personality research in the DSM-5 era. *Personality and Mental Health, 7*(3), 213–222. https://doi.org/10.1002/pmh.1217

Huprich, S. K. (2020). Personality disorders in the ICD-11: Opportunities and challenges for advancing the diagnosis of personality pathology. *Current Psychiatry Reports, 22*(8), 40. https://doi.org/10.1007/s11920-020-01161-4

Huprich, S. K., Herpertz, S. C., Bohus, M., Chanen, A. M., Goodman, M., Mehlum, L., Moran, P., Newton-Howe, G., Scott, L., & Sharp, C. (2018). Comment on Hopwood et al., "the time has come for dimensional personality disorder diagnosis." *Personality and Mental Health, 12*(1), 87–88.

Hurvich, M. (1970). On the concept of reality testing. *The International Journal of Psychoanalysis, 51*(3), 299–312.

Hutsebaut, J., Debbané, M., & Sharp, C. (2020). Designing a range of mentalizing interventions for young people using a clinical staging approach to borderline pathology. *Borderline Personality Disorder and Emotion Dysregulation, 7*(1), 6. https://doi.org/10.1186/s40479-020-0121-4

Hutsebaut, J., Weekers, L. C., Tuin, N., Apeldoorn, J. S. P., & Bulten, E. (2021). Assessment of ICD-11 personality disorder severity in forensic patients using the semi-structured interview for personality functioning DSM-5 (STiP-5.1): Preliminary findings. *Frontiers in Psychiatry, 12.* https://doi.org/10.3389/fpsyt.2021.617702

Hutsebaut, J. (2023). Isn't criterion A rather than B the language of psychotherapy?: Comment on Sauer-Zavala et al. (2022). *Personality Disorders: Theory, Research, and Treatment, 14*(4), 385–387. https://doi.org/10.1037/per0000543

Hyland, P., Karatzias, T., Shevlin, M., McElroy, E., Ben-Ezra, M., Cloitre, M., & Brewin, C. R. (2021). Does requiring trauma exposure affect rates of ICD-11 PTSD and complex PTSD? Implications for DSM–5. *Psychological Trauma: Theory, Research, Practice, and Policy, 13*(2), 133–141. https://doi.org/10.1037/tra0000908

Isaksson, J., Van't Westeinde, A., Cauvet, É., Kuja-Halkola, R., Lundin, K., Neufeld, J., Willfors, C., & Bölte, S. (2019). Social cognition in autism and other neurodevelopmental disorders: A co-twin control study. *Journal of Autism and Developmental Disorders, 49*(7), 2838–2848. https://doi.org/10.1007/s10803-019-04001-4

Jadav, N., & Bal, V. H. (2022). Associations between co-occurring conditions and age of autism diagnosis: Implications for mental health training and adult autism research. *Autism Research, 15*(11), 2112–2125. https://doi.org/10.1002/aur.2808

Johansen, M., Karterud, S., Pedersen, G., Gude, T., & Falkum, E. (2004). An investigation of the prototype validity of the borderline DSM-IV construct. *Acta Psychiatrica Scandinavica, 109*(4), 289–298. https://doi.org/10.1046/j.1600-0447.2003.00268.x

Jørgensen, C. R. (2006). Disturbed sense of identity in borderline personality disorder. *Journal of Personality Disorders, 20*(6), 618–644. https://doi.org/10.1521/pedi.2006.20.6.618

Jørgensen, C. R., Rasmussen, A. S., & Bøye, R. (2024). Level of identity diffusion in patients with borderline, narcissistic, avoidant and other specified personality disorder. *Nordic Psychology, 76*(3), 302–316. https://doi.org/10.1080/19012276.2023.2197561

Juul, S., Frandsen, F. W., Bo Hansen, S., Sørensen, P., Bateman, A., & Simonsen, S. (2022). A clinical illustration of short-term mentalization-based therapy for borderline personality disorder. *Journal of Clinical Psychology, 78*(8), 1567–1578. https://doi.org/10.1002/jclp.23378

Juul, S., Jakobsen, J. C., Hestbaek, E., Jørgensen, C. K., Olsen, M. H., Rishede, M., Frandsen, F. W., Bo, S., Lunn, S., Poulsen, S., Sørensen, P., Bateman, A., & Simonsen, S. (2023). Short-term versus long-term mentalization-based therapy for borderline personality disorder: A randomized clinical trial (MBT-RCT). *Psychotherapy and Psychosomatics, 92*(5), 329–339.

Karterud, S., Pedersen, G., Bjordal, E., Brabrand, J., Friis, S., Haaseth, Ø., Haavaldsen, G., Irion, T., Leirvåg, H., Tørum, E., & Urnes, Ø. (2003). Day treatment of patients with personality disorders: Experiences from a Norwegian treatment research network. *Journal of Personality Disorders, 17*(3), 243–262. https://doi.org/10.1521/pedi.17.3.243.22151

Karukivi, M., Vahlberg, T., Horjamo, K., Nevalainen, M., & Korkeila, J. (2017). Clinical importance of personality difficulties: Diagnostically sub-threshold personality disorders. *BMC Psychiatry, 17*(1), 16. https://doi.org/10.1186/s12888-017-1200-y

Kendler, K. S., Zachar, P., & Craver, C. (2011). What kinds of things are psychiatric disorders? *Psychological Medicine, 41*(6), 1143–1150. https://doi.org/10.1017/S0033291710001844

Kerber, A., Schultze, M., Müller, S., Rühling, R. M., Wright, A. G. C., Spitzer, C., Krueger, R. F., Knaevelsrud, C., & Zimmermann, J. (2022). Development of a short and ICD-11 compatible measure for DSM-5 maladaptive personality traits using ant colony optimization algorithms. *Assessment, 29*(3), 467–487.

Kernberg, O. F. (1967). Borderline personality organization. *Journal of the American Psychoanalytic Association, 15*(3), 641–685. https://doi.org/10.1177/000306516701500309

Kernberg, O. F. (2019). Psychotic personality structure. *Psychodynamic Psychiatry, 47*(4), 353–372. https://doi.org/10.1521/pdps.2019.47.4.353

Kiel, L., Hopwood, C. J., & Lind, M. (2024). Changes in personality functioning and pathological personality traits as a function of treatment: A feasibility study. *Journal of Psychopathology and Behavioral Assessment.* Advance online publication. https://doi.org/10.1007/s10862-024-10138-z

Kiel, L., Lind, M., & Spindler, H. (2024). What characterizes a well-functioning person? Perspectives from Scandinavian laypeople and mental health professionals. *Scandinavian Journal of Psychology.* Advance online publication. https://doi.org/10.1111/sjop.13041

Kiesler, D. J. (1986). The 1982 interpersonal circle: An analysis of DSM-III personality disorders. In T. Millon & G. L. Klerman (Eds.), *Contemporary directions in psychopathology: Toward the DSM-IV* (pp. 571–597). Guilford Press.

Kim, Y.-R., Blashfield, R. K., Tyrer, P., Hwang, S.-T., & Lee, H.-S. (2014). Field trial of a putative research algorithm for diagnosing ICD-11 personality disorders in psychiatric patients: 1. Severity of personality disturbance. *Personality and Mental Health, 8*(1), 67–78. https://doi.org/10.1002/pmh.1248

Kim, Y.-R., Tyrer, P., & Hwang, S. (2021). Personality Assessment Questionnaire for ICD-11 personality trait domains: Development and testing. *Personality and Mental Health, 15*(1), 58–71. https://doi.org/10.1002/pmh.1493

Kim, Y.-R., Tyrer, P., Lee, H.-S., Kim, S.-G., Connan, F., Kinnaird, E., Olajide, K., & Crawford, M. (2016). Schedule for personality assessment from notes and documents (SPAN-DOC): Preliminary validation, links to the ICD-11 classification of personality disorder, and use in eating disorders. *Personality and Mental Health, 10*(2), 106–117. https://doi.org/10.1002/pmh.1335

Kim, Y.-R., Tyrer, P., Lee, H.-S., Kim, S.-G., Hwang, S.-T., Lee, G. I. Y., & Mulder, R. T. (2015). Preliminary field trial of a putative research algorithm for diagnosing ICD-11 personality disorders in psychiatric patients: 2. Proposed trait domains. *Personality and Mental Health, 9*(4), 298–307.

Kongerslev, M. T., Chanen, A. M., & Simonsen, E. (2015). Personality disorder in childhood and adolescence comes of age: A review of the current evidence and prospects for future research. *Scandinavian Journal of Child and Adolescent Psychiatry and Psychology, 3*(1), 31–48. https://doi.org/10.21307/sjcapp-2015-004

Lavender, J. M., Wonderlich, S. A., Crosby, R. D., Engel, S. G., Mitchell, J. E., Crow, S. J., Peterson, C. B., & Le Grange, D. (2013). Personality-based subtypes of anorexia nervosa: Examining validity and utility using baseline clinical variables and ecological momentary assessment. *Behaviour Research and Therapy, 51*(8), 512–517. https://doi.org/10.1016/j.brat.2013.05.007

Ledden, S., Rains, L. S., Schlief, M., Barnett, P., Ching, B. C. F., Hallam, B., Günak, M. M., Steare, T., Parker, J., Labovitch, S., Oram, S., Pilling, S., Johnson, S., Papamichail, A., Mason, A., Thayaparan, A., Wang, B., Locke, C. D., Harju-Seppänen, J., … Haime, Z. (2022). Current state of the evidence on community treatments for people with complex emotional needs: A scoping review. *BMC Psychiatry, 22*(1), 589.

Lind, M., Adler, J. M., & Clark, L. A. (2020). Narrative identity and personality disorder: An empirical and conceptual review. *Current Psychiatry Reports, 22*(12), 67. https://doi.org/10.1007/s11920-020-01187-8

Linehan, M. M. (1993). *Cognitive-behavioral treatment of borderline personality disorder*. Guilford Press.

Linehan, M. M., & Dexter-Mazza, E. T. (2008). Dialectical behavior therapy for borderline personality disorder. In D. H. Barlow (Ed.), *Clinical handbook of psychological disorders: A step-by-step treatment manual* (4th ed., pp. 365–420). Guilford Press.

Lorentzen, H. S., Bårdsen, P. M., & Thimm, J. C. (2024). Reliability and validity of the Personality Disorder Severity ICD-11 (PDS-ICD-11) scale and the Revised Personality Assessment Questionnaire for ICD-11 (PAQ-11R) in a Norwegian community sample. *Personality and Mental Health.* https://doi.org/10.1002/pmh.1630

Lotfi, M., Bach, B., Amini, M., & Simonsen, E. (2018). Structure of DSM-5 and ICD-11 personality domains in Iranian community sample. *Personality and Mental Health, 12*(2), 155–169. https://doi.org/10.1002/pmh.1409

Lugo, V., de Oliveira, S. E. S., Hessel, C. R., Monteiro, R. T., Pasche, N. L., Pavan, G., Motta, L. S., Pacheco, M. A., & Spanemberg, L. (2019). Evaluation of DSM-5 and ICD-11 personality traits using the Personality Inventory for DSM-5 (PID-5) in a Brazilian sample of psychiatric inpatients. *Personality and Mental Health, 13*(1), 24–39. https://doi.org/10.1002/pmh.1436

Luyten, P., Campbell, C., Allison, E., & Fonagy, P. (2020). The mentalizing approach to psychopathology: State of the art and future directions. *Annual Review of Clinical Psychology, 16*(1), 297–325. https://doi.org/10.1146/annurev-clinpsy-071919-015355

Lynch, T. R., Hempel, R. J., & Dunkley, C. (2015). Radically open-dialectical behavior therapy for disorders of over-control: Signaling matters. *American Journal of Psychotherapy, 69*(2), 141–162. https://doi.org/10.1176/appi.psychotherapy.2015.69.2.141

Matthies, S., & Philipsen, A. (2016). Comorbidity of personality disorders and adult attention deficit hyperactivity disorder (ADHD): Review of recent findings. *Current Psychiatry Reports, 18*(4), 33. https://doi.org/10.1007/s11920-016-0675-4

McAdams, D. P. (2020). Psychopathology and the self: Human actors, agents, and authors. *Journal of Personality, 88*(1), 146–155. https://doi.org/10.1111/jopy.12496

McCrae, R. R. (1991). The five-factor model and its assessment in clinical settings. *Journal of Personality Assessment, 57*(3), 399–414. https://doi.org/10.1207/s15327752jpa5703_2

McLaren, V., Gallagher, M., Hopwood, C. J., & Sharp, C. (2022). Hypermentalizing and borderline personality disorder: A meta-analytic review. *American Journal of Psychotherapy, 75*(1), 21–31. https://doi.org/10.1176/appi.psychotherapy.20210018

McMain, S. F., Chapman, A. L., Kuo, J. R., Dixon-Gordon, K. L., Guimond, T. H., Labrish, C., Isaranuwatchai, W., & Streiner, D. L. (2022). The effectiveness of 6 versus 12 months of dialectical behavior therapy for borderline personality disorder: A noninferiority randomized clinical trial. *Psychotherapy and Psychosomatics, 91*(6), 382–397. https://doi.org/10.1159/000525102

Miller, T. W. (1991). The psychotherapeutic utility of the five-factor model of personality: A clinician's experience. *Journal of Personality Assessment, 57*(3), 415–433. https://doi.org/10.1207/s15327752jpa5703_3

Morey, L. C. (2017). Development and initial evaluation of a self-report form of the DSM-5 Level of Personality Functioning Scale. *Psychological Assessment, 29*(10), 1302–1308. https://doi.org/10.1037/pas0000450

Morey, L. C., & Hopwood, C. J. (2019). Expert preferences for categorical, dimensional, and mixed/hybrid approaches to personality disorder diagnosis. *Journal of Personality Disorders*, 34(Suppl. C), 124–131. https://doi.org/10.1521/pedi_2019_33_398

Morgan, T. A., Chelminski, I., Young, D., Dalrymple, K., & Zimmerman, M. (2013). Is dimensional scoring important only for subthreshold levels of severity in personality disorders other than borderline? *Comprehensive Psychiatry, 54*(6), 673–679. https://doi.org/10.1016/j.comppsych.2013.01.008

Moselli, M., Casini, M. P., Frattini, C., & Williams, R. (2023). Suicidality and personality pathology in adolescence: A systematic review. *Child Psychiatry & Human Development, 54*(2), 290–311. https://doi.org/10.1007/s10578-021-01239-x

Mulder, R. T., Horwood, J., Tyrer, P., Carter, J., & Joyce, P. R. (2016). Validating the proposed ICD-11 domains. *Personality and Mental Health, 10*(2), 84–95. https://doi.org/10.1002/pmh.1336

Mulder, R. T., Newton-Howes, G., Crawford, M. J., & Tyrer, P. (2011). The central domains of personality pathology in psychiatric patients. *Journal of Personality Disorders, 25*(3), 364–377. https://doi.org/10.1521/pedi.2011.25.3.364

Mulder, R. T., & Tyrer, P. (2023). Borderline personality disorder: A spurious condition unsupported by science that should be abandoned. *Journal of the Royal Society of Medicine, 116*(4), 148–150. https://doi.org/10.1177/01410768231164780

Müller, K. W., Dreier, M., & Wölfling, K. (2023). Personality traits and their role as risk modifiers in gaming disorder and internet use disorders. *Current Opinion in Psychiatry, 36*(1), 75–79. https://doi.org/10.1097/YCO.0000000000000827

Navarro-Gómez, S., Frías, Á., & Palma, C. (2017). Romantic relationships of people with borderline personality: A narrative review. *Psychopathology, 50*(3), 175–187. https://doi.org/10.1159/000474950

Newton-Howes, G., Tyrer, P., Johnson, T., Mulder, R. T., Kool, S., Dekker, J., & Schoevers, R. (2014). Influence of personality on the outcome of treatment in depression: Systematic review and meta-analysis. *Journal of Personality Disorders, 28*(4), 577–593. https://doi.org/10.1521/pedi_2013_27_070

Ohi, K., Shimada, T., Nitta, Y., Kihara, H., Okubo, H., Uehara, T., & Kawasaki, Y. (2016). The five-factor model personality traits in schizophrenia: A meta-analysis. *Psychiatry Research, 240*, 34–41. https://doi.org/10.1016/j.psychres.2016.04.004

Oltmanns, J. R., & Widiger, T. A. (2018). A self-report measure for the ICD-11 dimensional trait model proposal: The Personality Inventory for ICD-11. *Psychological Assessment, 30*(2), 154–169. https://doi.org/10.1037/pas0000459

Oltmanns, J. R., & Widiger, T. A. (2020). The Five-Factor Personality Inventory for ICD-11: A facet-level assessment of the ICD-11 trait model. *Psychological Assessment, 32*(1), 60–71. https://doi.org/10.1037/pas0000763

Oltmanns, J. R., & Widiger, T. A. (2021). The self- and informant-personality inventories for ICD-11: Agreement, structure, and relations with health, social, and satisfaction variables in older adults. *Psychological Assessment, 33*(4), 300–310. https://doi.org/10.1037/pas0000982

Pan, B., & Wang, W. (2024). Practical implications of ICD-11 personality disorder classifications. *BMC Psychiatry, 24*(1), Article 191.

Paret, C., Jennen-Steinmetz, C., & Schmahl, C. (2017). Disadvantageous decision-making in borderline personality disorder: Partial support from a meta-analytic review. *Neuroscience & Biobehavioral Reviews, 72*, 301–309. https://doi.org/10.1016/j.neubiorev.2016.11.019

Paris, J. (2015). *Overdiagnosis in psychiatry: How modern psychiatry lost its way while creating a diagnosis for almost all of life's misfortunes* (1st ed.). Oxford University Press. https://doi.org/10.1093/med/9780199350643.001.0001

Pedersen, L., & Simonsen, E. (2014). Incidence and prevalence rates of personality disorders in Denmark: A register study. *Nordic Journal of Psychiatry, 68*(8), 543–548. https://doi.org/10.3109/08039488.2014.884630

Peter, L.-J., Schindler, S., Sander, C., Schmidt, S., Muehlan, H., McLaren, T., Tomczyk, S., Speerforck, S., & Schomerus, G. (2021). Continuum beliefs and mental illness stigma: A systematic review and meta-analysis of correlation and intervention studies. *Psychological Medicine, 51*(5), 716–726. https://doi.org/10.1055/s-0041-1732168

Prevolnik Rupel, V., Jagger, B., Fialho, L. S., Chadderton, L.-M., Gintner, T., Arntz, A., Baltzersen, Å.-L., Blazdell, J., van Busschbach, J., Cencelli, M., Chanen, A., Delvaux, C., van Gorp, F., Langford, L., McKenna, B., Moran, P., Pacheco, K., Sharp, C., Wang, W., … Crawford, M. J. (2021). Standard set of patient-reported outcomes for personality disorder. *Quality of Life Research, 30*(12), 3485–3500.

Pull, C. B. (2014). Personality disorders in Diagnostic and Statistical Manual of Mental Disorders-5. *Current Opinion in Psychiatry, 27*(1), 84–86. https://doi.org/10.1097/YCO.0000000000000016

Reed, G. M. (2010). Toward ICD-11: Improving the clinical utility of WHO's international classification of mental disorders. *Professional Psychology: Research and Practice, 41*(6), 457–464. https://doi.org/10.1037/a0021701

Reed, G. M. (2018). Progress in developing a classification of personality disorders for ICD-11. *World Psychiatry, 17*(2), 227–228. https://doi.org/10.1002/wps.20533

Reed, G. M. (2024). What's in a name? Mental disorders, mental health conditions and psychosocial disability. *World Psychiatry, 23*(2), 209–210. https://doi.org/10.1002/wps.21190

Reed, G. M., Correia, J. M., Esparza, P., Saxena, S., & Maj, M. (2011). The WPA–WHO global survey of psychiatrists' attitudes towards mental disorders classification. *World Psychiatry, 10*(2), 118–131. https://doi.org/10.1002/j.2051-5545.2011.tb00034.x

Ricoeur, P. (1992). *Oneself as another*. University of Chicago Press.

Rinaldi, C., Attanasio, M., Valenti, M., Mazza, M., & Keller, R. (2021). Autism spectrum disorder and personality disorders: Comorbidity and differential diagnosis. *World Journal of Psychiatry, 11*(12), 1366–1386. https://doi.org/10.5498/wjp.v11.i12.1366

Roche, M. J. (2018). Examining the alternative model for personality disorder in daily life: Evidence for incremental validity. *Personality Disorder: Theory, Research, and Treatment, 9*(6), 574–583. https://doi.org/10.1037/per0000295

Ronningstam, E., & Baskin-Sommers, A. R. (2013). Fear and decision-making in narcissistic personality disorder: A link between psychoanalysis and neuroscience. *Dialogues in Clinical Neuroscience, 15*(2), 191–201. https://doi.org/10.31887/DCNS.2013.15.2/eronningstam

Rubæk, L., & Møhl, B. (2023). Direct and indirect self-injury. In E. Lloyd-Richardson, I. Baetens, & J. Whitlock (Eds.), *The Oxford Handbook of Nonsuicidal Self-Injury* (pp. 41–71). Oxford University Press. https://doi.org/10.1093/oxfordhb/9780197611272.013.4

Sahin, Z., Vinnars, B., Gorman, B. S., Wilczek, A., Åsberg, M., & Barber, J. P. (2018). Clinical severity as a moderator of outcome in psychodynamic and dialectical behavior therapies for borderline personality disorder. *Personality Disorders: Theory, Research, and Treatment, 9*(5), 437–446. https://doi.org/10.1037/per0000276

Samuel, D. B., & Widiger, T. A. (2007). Describing Ted Bundy's personality and working towards DSM-V. *Independent Practitioner, 27*(1), 20–22.

Saulsman, L. M., & Page, A. C. (2004). The five-factor model and personality disorder empirical literature: A meta-analytic review. *Clinical Psychology Review, 23*(8), 1055–1085. https://doi.org/10.1016/j.cpr.2002.09.001

Scott, C., & Medeiros, M. (2020). Personality and political careers: What personality types are likely to run for office and get elected? *Personality and Individual Differences, 152*, 109600. https://doi.org/10.1016/j.paid.2019.109600

Sebastian, A., Jacob, G., Lieb, K., & Tüscher, O. (2013). Impulsivity in borderline personality disorder: A matter of disturbed impulse control or a facet of emotional dysregulation? *Current Psychiatry Reports, 15*(2), 339. https://doi.org/10.1007/s11920-012-0339-y

Sellbom, M., Bach, B., & Huxley, E. (2018). Related personality disorders located within an elaborated externalizing psychopathology spectrum. In J. E. Lochman & W. Matthys (Eds.), *The Wiley handbook of disruptive and impulse-control disorders* (pp. 103–124). Wiley & Sons.

Sellbom, M., Brown, T. A., & Bach, B. (2024). Development and psychometric evaluation of the Personality Disorder Severity ICD-11 (PDS-ICD-11) clinician-rating form. *Personality and Mental Health, 18*(1), 60–68. https://doi.org/10.1002/pmh.1596

Sellbom, M., Chiasson, P. M., Brown, T. A., & Bach, B. (2023). Examining the construct validity of the Personality Assessment Questionnaire for ICD-11 (PAQ-11) personality trait domains in a community sample. *Personality and Mental Health, 17*(3), 197–207. https://doi.org/10.1002/pmh.1573

Sellbom, M., Solomon-Krakus, S., Bach, B., & Bagby, R. M. (2020). Validation of Personality Inventory for DSM-5 (PID-5) algorithms to assess ICD-11 personality trait domains in a psychiatric sample. *Psychological Assessment, 32*(1), 40–49. https://doi.org/10.1037/pas0000746

Sharp, C. (2018). Calling for a unified redefinition of "borderlineness": Commentary on Gunderson et al. *Journal of Personality Disorders, 32*(2), 168–174. https://doi.org/10.1521/pedi.2018.32.2.168

Sharp, C., & Oldham, J. (2023). Nature and assessment of personality pathology and diagnosis. *American Journal of Psychotherapy, 76*(1), 3–8. https://doi.org/10.1176/appi.psychotherapy.20220016

Sharp, C., & Wall, K. (2021). DSM-5 level of personality functioning: Refocusing personality disorder on what it means to be human. *Annual Review of Clinical Psychology, 17*(1), 313–337. https://doi.org/10.1146/annurev-clinpsy-081219-105402

Simon, J., & Bach, B. (2022). Organization of clinician-rated personality disorder types according to ICD-11 severity of personality dysfunction. *Psychodynamic Psychiatry, 50*(4), 672–688. https://doi.org/10.1521/pdps.2022.50.4.672

Simon, J., Lambrecht, B., & Bach, B. (2023). Cross-walking personality disorder types to ICD-11 trait domains: An overview of current findings. *Frontiers in Psychiatry, 14*. https://doi.org/10.3389/fpsyt.2023.1175425

Simonsen, E., & Newton-Howes, G. (2018). Personality pathology and schizophrenia. *Schizophrenia Bulletin, 44*(6), 1180–1184. https://doi.org/10.1093/schbul/sby053

Simonsen, S., Bateman, A. W., Bohus, M., Dalewijk, H. J., Doering, S., Kaera, A., Moran, P., Renneberg, B., Ribaudi, J. S., Taubner, S., Wilberg, T., & Mehlum, L. (2019). European guidelines for personality disorders: Past, present and future. *Borderline Personality Disorder and Emotion Dysregulation, 6*(1), 9. https://doi.org/10.1186/s40479-019-0106-3

Simonsen, S., Eikenaes, I. U.-M., Bach, B., Kvarstein, E., Gondan, M., Møller, S. B., & Wilberg, T. (2021). Level of alexithymia as a measure of personality dysfunction in avoidant personality disorder. *Nordic Journal of Psychiatry, 75*(4), 266–274. https://doi.org/10.1080/08039488.2020.1841290

Simonsen, S., Heinskou, T., Sørensen, P., Folke, S., & Lau, M. E. (2017). Personality disorders: Patient characteristics and level of outpatient treatment service. *Nordic Journal of Psychiatry, 71*(5), 325–331. https://doi.org/10.1080/08039488.2017.1284262

Simonsen, S., Popolo, R., Juul, S., Frandsen, F. W., Sørensen, P., & Dimaggio, G. (2022). Treating avoidant personality disorder with combined individual metacognitive interpersonal therapy and group mentalization-based treatment. *Journal of Nervous & Mental Disease, 210*(3), 163–171. https://doi.org/10.1097/NMD.0000000000001432

Skodol, A. E. (2014). Manifestations, assessment, and differential diagnosis. In J. M. Oldham, A. E. Skodol, & D. S. Bender (Eds.), *The American Psychiatric Association Publishing textbook of personality disorders* (2nd ed., pp. 131–164). American Psychiatric Association Publishing.

Skodol, A. E., Morey, L. C., Bender, D. S., & Oldham, J. M. (2013). When is it time to move on? Rejoinder for "The ironic fate of the personality disorders in DSM-5." *Personality Disorders: Theory, Research, and Treatment, 4*(4), 354–354. https://doi.org/10.1037/per0000054

Sletved, K. S. O., Villemoes, N. H. F., Coello, K., Stanislaus, S., Kjærstad, H. L., Faurholt-Jepsen, M., Miskowiak, K., Bukh, J. D., Vinberg, M., & Kessing, L. V. (2023). Personality disorders in patients with newly diagnosed bipolar disorder, their unaffected first-degree relatives and healthy control individuals. *Journal of Affective Disorders, 327*, 183–189.

Smith, D. J., Muir, W. J., & Blackwood, D. H. R. (2004). Is borderline personality disorder part of the bipolar spectrum? *Harvard Review of Psychiatry, 12*(3), 133–139. https://doi.org/10.1080/10673220490472346

Smith, T. E., & Samuel, D. B. (2017). A multi-method examination of the links between ADHD and personality disorder. *Journal of Personality Disorders, 31*(1), 26–48. https://doi.org/10.1521/pedi_2016_30_236

Soeteman, D. I., Verheul, R., & Bussehbaeh, J. J. V. (2008). The burden of disease in personality disorders: Diagnosis-specific quality of life. *Journal of Personality Disorders, 22*(3), 259–268. https://doi.org/10.1521/pedi.2008.22.3.259

Solbakken, O. A., Hansen, R. S., & Monsen, J. T. (2011). Affect integration and reflective function: Clarification of central conceptual issues. *Psychotherapy Research, 21*(4), 482–496. https://doi.org/10.1080/10503307.2011.583696

Sorrel, M. A., Aluja, A., García, L. F., & Gutiérrez, F. (2022). Psychometric properties of the Five-Factor Personality Inventory for ICD-11 (FFiCD) in Spanish community samples. *Psychological Assessment, 34*(3), 281–293. https://doi.org/10.1037/pas0001084

Speed, B. C., Goldstein, B. L., & Goldfried, M. R. (2018). Assertiveness training: A forgotten evidence-based treatment. *Clinical Psychology: Science and Practice, 25*(1).

Storebø, O. J., & Simonsen, E. (2014). Is ADHD an early stage in the development of borderline personality disorder? *Nordic Journal of Psychiatry, 68*(5), 289–295. https://doi.org/10.3109/08039488.2013.841992

Storebø, O. J., Stoffers-Winterling, J. M., Völlm, B. A., Kongerslev, M. T., Mattivi, J. T., Jørgensen, M. S., Faltinsen, E., Todorovac, A., Sales, C. P., Callesen, H. E., Lieb, K., & Simonsen, E. (2020). Psychological therapies for people with borderline personality disorder. *Cochrane Database of Systematic Reviews, 5*(5), CD012955. https://doi.org/10.1002/14651858.CD012955.pub2

Stricker, J., Hasenburg, L., Jakob, L., Weigl, T., & Pietrowsky, R. (2024). Public stigma and continuum beliefs across personality disorder severity levels. *Journal of Personality Disorders, 38*(1), 75–86. https://doi.org/10.1521/pedi.2024.38.1.75

Sullivan, H. S. (1968). *The interpersonal theory of psychiatry*. W. W. Norton.

Swales, M. A. (2022). Personality disorder diagnoses in ICD-11: Transforming conceptualisations and practice [Special issue]. *Clinical Psychology in Europe, 4*. https://doi.org/10.32872/cpe.9635

Taylor, C. (1989). *Sources of the self: The making of the modern identity*. Harvard University Press.

Taylor, G. J., & Bagby, R. M. (2012). The Alexithymia Personality Dimension. In T. A. Widiger (Ed.), *The Oxford handbook of personality disorders* (pp. 647–673). Oxford University Press.

Tiger, A., Ohlis, A., Bjureberg, J., Lundström, S., Lichtenstein, P., Larsson, H., Hellner, C., Kuja-Halkola, R., & Jayaram-Lindström, N. (2022). Childhood symptoms of attention-deficit/hyperactivity disorder and borderline personality disorder. *Acta Psychiatrica Scandinavica, 146*(4), 370–380. https://doi.org/10.1111/acps.13476

Traynor, J. M., McMain, S., Chapman, A. L., Kuo, J., Labrish, C., & Ruocco, A. C. (2024). Pretreatment cognitive performance is associated with differential self-harm outcomes in 6 v. 12-months of dialectical behavior therapy for borderline personality disorder. *Psychological Medicine, 54*(7), 1350–1360. https://doi.org/10.1017/S0033291723003197

Tseng, S., & Georgiades, A. (2024). A phenomenological comparison of auditory hallucinations between borderline personality disorder and schizophrenia: A systematic review. *Clinical Psychology & Psychotherapy, 31*(1). https://doi.org/10.1002/cpp.2958

Tyrer, P. (2002). Nidotherapy: A new approach to the treatment of personality disorder. *Acta Psychiatrica Scandinavica, 105*(6), 469–471. https://doi.org/10.1034/j.1600-0447.2002.01362.x

Tyrer, P. (2005). The problem of severity in the classification of personality disorder. *Journal of Personality Disorders, 19*(3), 309–314. https://doi.org/10.1521/pedi.2005.19.3.309

Tyrer, P., & Alexander, J. (1979). Classification of personality disorder. *British Journal of Psychiatry, 135*(2), 163–167. https://doi.org/10.1192/bjp.135.2.163

Tyrer, P., Crawford, M., & Mulder, R. T. (2011). Reclassifying personality disorders. *The Lancet, 377*(9780), 1814–1815.

Tyrer, P., Crawford, M., Mulder, R. T., Blashfield, R. K., Farnam, A., Fossati, A., Kim, Y.-R., Koldobsky, N., Lecic-Tosevski, D., Ndetei, D., Swales, M., Clark, L. A., & Reed, G. M. (2011). The rationale for the reclassification of personality disorder in the 11th revision of the International Classification of Diseases (ICD-11). *Personality and Mental Health, 5*(4), 246–259.

Tyrer, P., Crawford, M., Sanatinia, R., Tyrer, H., Cooper, S., Muller-Pollard, C., Christodoulou, P., Zauter-Tutt, M., Miloseska-Reid, K. K., Loebenberg, G., Guo, B., Yang, M., Wang, D., & Weich, S. (2014). Preliminary studies of the ICD-11 classification of personality disorder in practice. *Personality and Mental Health, 8*(4), 254–263.

Tyrer, P., & Johnson, T. (1996). Establishing the severity of personality disorder. *American Journal of Psychiatry, 153*(12), 1593–1597. https://doi.org/10.1176/ajp.153.12.1593

Tyrer, P., Mulder, R. T., Kim, Y.-R., & Crawford, M. J. (2019). The development of the ICD-11 classification of personality disorders: An amalgam of science, pragmatism, and politics. *Annual Review of Clinical Psychology, 15*(1), 481–502. https://doi.org/10.1146/annurev-clinpsy-050718-095736

Tyrer, P., Mulder, R. T., Newton-Howes, G., & Duggan, C. (2022). Galenic syndromes: Combinations of mental state and personality disorders too closely entwined to be separated. *British Journal of Psychiatry, 220*(6), 309–310. https://doi.org/10.1192/bjp.2021.220

Tyrer, P., Reed, G. M., & Crawford, M. J. (2015). Classification, assessment, prevalence, and effect of personality disorder. *The Lancet, 385*(9969), 717–726.

Vegni, N., D'Ardia, C., & Torregiani, G. (2021). Empathy, mentalization, and theory of mind in borderline personality disorder: Possible overlap with autism spectrum disorders. *Frontiers in Psychology, 12*. https://doi.org/10.3389/fpsyg.2021.626353

Verheul, R. (2001). Co-morbidity of personality disorders in individuals with substance use disorders. *European Psychiatry, 16*, 274–282. https://doi.org/10.1016/S0924-9338(01)00578-8

Villemarette-Pittman, N. R., Stanford, M. S., Greve, K. W., Houston, R. J., & Mathias, C. W. (2004). Obsessive-compulsive personality disorder and behavioral disinhibition. *The Journal of Psychology, 138*(1), 5–22.

Volkert, J., Gablonski, T.-C., & Rabung, S. (2018). Prevalence of personality disorders in the general adult population in Western countries: Systematic review and meta-analysis. *British Journal of Psychiatry, 213*(6), 709–715. https://doi.org/10.1192/bjp.2018.202

Weekers, L. C., Hutsebaut, J., & Kamphuis, J. H. (2019). The Level of Personality Functioning Scale-Brief Form 2.0: Update of a brief instrument for assessing level of personality functioning. *Personality and Mental Health, 13*(1), 3–14.

Weekers, L. C., Hutsebaut, J., Rovers, J. M. C., & Kamphuis, J. H. (2024). Head-to-head comparison of the alternative model for personality disorders and section II personality disorder model in terms of predicting patient outcomes 1 year later. *Personality Disorders: Theory, Research, and Treatment, 15*(2), 101–109. https://doi.org/10.1037/per0000637

Weiss, R. D., & Mirin, S. M. (1986). Subtypes of cocaine abusers. *Psychiatric Clinics of North America, 9*(3), 491–501. https://doi.org/10.1016/S0193-953X(18)30608-7

Widiger, T. A. (2011). Personality and psychopathology. *World Psychiatry, 10*(2), 103–106. https://doi.org/10.1002/j.2051-5545.2011.tb00024.x

Widiger, T. A., & Crego, C. (2019). The Five Factor Model of personality structure: An update. *World Psychiatry, 18*(3), 271–272. https://doi.org/10.1002/wps.20658

Widiger, T. A., Hines, A., & Crego, C. (2024). Evidence-based assessment of personality disorder. *Assessment, 31*(1), 191–198. https://doi.org/10.1177/10731911231176461

Widiger, T. A., & Oltmanns, J. R. (2017). Neuroticism is a fundamental domain of personality with enormous public health implications. *World Psychiatry, 16*(2), 144–145. https://doi.org/10.1002/wps.20411

Widiger, T. A., & Simonsen, E. (2005). Alternative dimensional models of personality disorder: Finding a common ground. *Journal of Personality Disorders, 19*(2), 110–130. https://doi.org/10.1521/pedi.19.2.110.62628

Widiger, T. A., & Trull, T. J. (1992). Personality and psychopathology: An application of the five-factor model. *Journal of Personality, 60*(2), 363–393. https://doi.org/10.1111/j.1467-6494.1992.tb00977.x

World Health Organization. (1992). *The ICD-10 classification of mental and behavioural disorders: clinical descriptions and diagnostic guidelines*. World Health Organization.

World Health Organization. (2024). *Clinical descriptions and diagnostic requirements for ICD-11 mental, behavioural and neurodevelopmental disorders*. World Health Organization.

Widiger, T. A., & Trull, T. J. (2007). Plate tectonics in the classification of personality disorder. *American Psychologist, 62*, 71–83. https://doi.org/10.1037/0003-066X.62.2.71

Wilson, S., Stroud, C. B., & Durbin, C. E. (2017). Interpersonal dysfunction in personality disorders: A meta-analytic review. *Psychological Bulletin, 143*(7), 677–734. https://doi.org/10.1037/bul0000101

Wright, A. G. C., Hopwood, C. J., Skodol, A. E., & Morey, L. C. (2016). Longitudinal validation of general and specific structural features of personality pathology. *Journal of Abnormal Psychology, 125*(8), 1120–1134. https://doi.org/10.1037/abn0000165

Yang, M., Coid, J., & Tyrer, P. (2010). Personality pathology recorded by severity: National survey. *British Journal of Psychiatry, 197*(3), 193–199. https://doi.org/10.1192/bjp.bp.110.078956

Young, J. E., Klosko, J. S., & Weishaar, M. E. (2003). *Schema therapy: A practitioner's guide*. Guilford Press.

Zandersen, M., & Parnas, J. (2018). Identity disturbance, feelings of emptiness, and the boundaries of the schizophrenia spectrum. *Schizophrenia Bulletin, 45*(January), 106–113.

Zandersen, M., & Parnas, J. (2019). Borderline personality disorder or a disorder within the schizophrenia spectrum? A psychopathological study. *World Psychiatry, 18*(1), 109–110. https://doi.org/10.1002/wps.20598

Zimmerman, M., Chelminski, I., Young, D., Dalrymple, K., & Martinez, J. (2013). Is dimensional scoring of borderline personality disorder important only for subthreshold levels of severity? *Journal of Personality Disorders, 27*(2), 244–251. https://doi.org/10.1521/pedi_2012_26_022

Zimmermann, J., Falk, C. F., Wendt, L., Spitzer, C., Fischer, H. F., Bach, B., Sellbom, M., Müller, S., Fischer, F., Bach, B., Sellbom, M., & Müller, S. (2023). Validating the German version of the Personality Disorder Severity-ICD-11 scale using nominal response models. *Psychological Assessment, 35*(3), 257–268. https://doi.org/10.31234/osf.io/42whs

Zimmermann, J., Müller, S., Bach, B., Hutsebaut, J., Hummelen, B., & Fischer, F. (2020). A common metric for self-reported severity of personality disorder. *Psychopathology, 53*(3–4), 168–178. https://doi.org/10.1159/000507377

Appendix A
Assessment

Basically, any clinician across all World Health Organization member states should be able to diagnose a Personality Disorder using the ICD-11 clinical descriptions and diagnostic requirements without additional measures or instruments. Therefore, it should generally be possible for clinicians to determine the severity of a Personality Disorder based on clinical observations and other available information (e.g., medical records and information from relatives). However, standardised instruments can help ensure consistency and thoroughness in diagnosis (e.g., reliability). A number of scales, procedure, and instruments have already been developed, evaluated, and validated for ICD-11 Personality Disorders and Related Traits (Aydin-Seyrek et al., 2024; Hualparuca-Olivera, Caycho-Rodríguez et al., 2024; Bach & Mulder, 2022). We will now outline which instruments and options are currently available for both severity and trait domain assessment.

Severity Assessment

A Danish–New Zealand collaboration has led to the development of the Diagnostic Interview for Personality Pathology in ICD-11 (DIPP-11) for clinical assessment and diagnosis of ICD-11 Personality Disorders and Related Traits (Bach & Sellbom, 2025). The DIPP-11 interview is partially developed from the Personality Disorder Severity ICD-11 (PDS-ICD-11) scale, which exclusively measures disturbances in aspects of the self and interpersonal functioning along with emotional, cognitive, and behavioural manifestations, and global psychosocial impairment (Bach et al., 2021). Beyond the self-report form, the PDS-ICD-11 scale also exists as a clinician-rating form, which can be answered based on a clinical interview or based on adequate knowledge about the patient (Sellbom et al., 2024). The PDS-ICD-11 consists of 14 items (i.e., themes or questions) to be rated based on different statements that match different levels of severity. Prior to the development of the PDS-ICD-11, the Level of Personality Functioning Scale – Brief Form (LPFS-BF) was recommended to measure the severity of personality dysfunction according to ICD-11 (Prevolnik Rupel et al., 2021). In addition to the basic aspects of self and interpersonal functioning described in the LPFS-BF, the PDS-ICD-11 and the DIPP-11 also cover features such as reality testing (i.e., cognitive manifestations), harm to self and others (i.e., behavioural manifestations), and global psychosocial impairment.

So far, the PDS-ICD-11 scale has been evaluated in the US, New Zealand, Germany, Spain, Peru, Norway, and Denmark (Bach et al., 2023; Bach et al., 2021; Gutiérrez, Aluja, Rodríguez et al., 2022; Hualparuca-Olivera, Calle-Arancibia et al., 2024; Lorentzen et al., 2024; Zimmermann et al., 2023), and several international studies are currently underway. Overall, the research supports that the PDS-ICD-11 scale measures a global dimension of personality dysfunction. In addition, there is considerable agreement between the PDS-ICD-11 and other established measures of personality functioning, including the LPFS-BF, borderline symptom score, and a global Personality Disorder score based on DSM-5 criteria.

Crucially, a clinical sample from New Zealand found that the PDS-ICD-11 scale was useful in distinguishing between patients with and without a diagnosed Personality Disorder (Bach et al., 2021). Across the US, New Zealand, German, and Danish samples, it has been found that a score of approximately 16–17 indicates pronounced dysfunction. More specifically, in a Danish representative national sample (n = 3,044), it was found that cut-off values of 9, 12, 19, and 22 can be interpreted as indicating mild, moderate, severe, and extreme dysfunction, respectively (Bach et al., 2023). Findings from both the Danish sample and the Peruvian adolescent study suggest that these cut-off values should be significantly higher for younger people (Bach et al., 2023; Hualparuca-Olivera, Calle-Arancibia et al., 2024). Table A1 provides an overview of the themes uncovered by the PDS-ICD-11 according to healthy personality functioning. Both the self-report and clinician-rating forms of the PDS-ICD-11 scale are freely available and accessible with the published development studies (Bach et al., 2021; Sellbom et al., 2024). A number of international translations of the PDS-ICD-11 scales are also freely available.

Together with a local research team, Clark and colleagues (2021) developed a set of preliminary scales corresponding to the definitions of severity and the specific personality traits in the ICD-11. A total of 65 items included in this instrument are designed to uncover aspects of self and interpersonal functioning, including identity, self-esteem, self-perception, goal orientation, and relationships along with 181 other items that cover trait domains and facets. However, the emotional, cognitive, and behavioural manifestations as well as global psychosocial impairment are not covered by this instrument.

Table A1 Personality functioning in ICD-11 operationalised with the PDS-ICD-11 scale

Capabilities and manifestations	Healthy functioning
1. Identity	Stability and coherence of one's sense of identity (e.g., the extent to which identity or sense of self is variable and contradictory or overly rigid and fixed)
2. Self-esteem	Ability to maintain an overall positive and stable sense of self-worth
3. Self-perception	Realistic view of one's own capabilities, strengths, and limitations
4. Goals	Capacity for self-direction (ability to plan, select, and realise appropriate goals)
5. Interest in relationships	Has a good balance between being alone and being with others
6. Perspective-taking	Ability to understand and appreciate other people's perspectives without overthinking what they think and feel
7. Mutuality in relationships	Ability to develop and maintain close and mutually satisfying relationships
8. Disagreement management	Ability to manage conflict in relationships in a cooperative manner
9. Controlling and showing emotions	Ability to control and express own emotions in an appropriate way
10. Behavioural control	Ability to be spontaneous while having appropriate control over your actions
11. Experience of reality during stress	Realistic situational and interpersonal judgement, especially under stress
12. Harm to self 13. Harm to others	Appropriate behavioural response to intense emotions and stressful circumstances
14. Psychosocial impairment	Functioning in personal, family, social, educational, employment, and other important areas of life

Note. PDS-ICD-11 = Personality Disorder Severity ICD-11.

In addition to the aforementioned ICD-11 instruments, there are also a number of other instruments originally developed for the DSM-5 alternative model of Personality Disorders. So far, these tools have worked satisfactorily for estimating severity in a way that largely corresponds to certain aspects of the ICD-11 classification of Personality Disorder. These instruments include self-report tools such as the Self and Interpersonal Functioning Scale (Gamache et al., 2021), the LPFS-BF (Bach & Hutsebaut, 2018; Weekers et al., 2019), Level of Personality Functioning Scale – Self-Report (Morey, 2017), and Levels of Personality Functioning Questionnaire for Youth (Goth et al., 2018). The fact that these instruments basically overlap, supports that they can serve to describe the majority of the information needed to determine the severity of Personality Disorder according to ICD-11 (Zimmermann et al., 2020). However, they do not exhaustively capture all ICD-11 definitions, such as impaired reality testing and harm to self or others. Besides the afore-mentioned DSM-5 self-report instruments, the following DSM-5 interview-based instruments can also be said to generate the most important informa-tion for classification of severity according to ICD-11: the Semi-Structured Interview for DSM-5 Personality Functioning (Hutsebaut et al., 2021) and the Structured Clinical Interview for DSM-5 Alternative Model of Personal-ity Disorders (First et al., 2018).

Assessment of Trait Domains

As already described in Chapter 5 and Chapter 6, the specification of trait do-mains helps to characterise the individual expression of the Personality Dis-order, allowing the clinician to better understand the issues causing the dys-function that should be considered in clinical planning and treatment. For example, it makes a significant difference whether a patient with Moderate Personality Disorder is characterised by prominent Negative Affectivity and Anankastia (e.g., anxiousness and perfectionism) or prominent Dissociality and Disinhibition (e.g., lack of empathy, and risk-taking behaviour). Thus, two people with the same level of severity may need different interventions due to their different composition of trait domains. Assessment should there-fore consider both global severity of Personality Disorder and how individ-ual traits contribute to the expression of thereof.

At least six different instruments have been developed to measure and de-scribe personality traits in ICD-11. An overview of four of these instruments along with their subscales is presented in Table A2. The Personality Inven-tory for ICD-11 instrument consists of 60 items (Oltmanns & Widiger, 2018) and a corresponding Informant-Personality Inventory for ICD-11 is also available (Bach, Christensen et al., 2020; Oltmanns & Widiger, 2021). The use of both instruments has been supported in a number of studies. For clinicians or researchers who need a quick assessment or screening, there is the Personality Assessment Questionnaire for ICD-11 personality traits, which consists of only 17 items (Kim et al., 2021; Sellbom et al., 2023). The Personality Inventory for DSM-5 and ICD-11 Plus Modified is available in a 30-item version that effectively and exclusively describes the five ICD-11 trait domains and 15 subscales (Bach, Kerber, et al., 2020; Kerber et al., 2022). This instrument has demonstrated robust psychometric properties across more than 12 languages. For clinicians who desire a more fine-grained and clinically informative portrayal of personality traits, the Five-Factor Inventory for ICD-11 measures not only the five domains, but also 20 facets (e.g., anxiousness, self-centredness) and 47 nuances (e.g., separation anxiety, vanity) based on 121 items (Oltmanns & Widiger, 2020). For clinicians already using the well-established Personality Inventory for DSM-5, there is an algorithm to describe the ICD-11 domains as well as 18 clinically informative subscales (Bach et al., 2017; Sellbom et al., 2020), which have been evaluated in a number of international studies (e.g., Hemmati et al., 2021; Lotfi et al., 2018; Lugo et al., 2019). Most recently, Clark and colleagues (2021) developed and evaluated a set of preliminary scales for ICD-11 personality traits, based on 151 items describing the five domains with 11 facet-like subscales. Tables A2 and A3 provide an overview of four of the instruments, which also portray facets and nuances in the form of subscales.

Table A2   Four models for describing trait domains and facets in ICD-11

	FFiCD	PID-5 algorithm	Clark et al. scales	PID5BF+M
No. of items	121 items	158 items	181 items	30 items
Negative Affectivity	Emotional lability	Emotional lability	Emotional lability	Emotional lability
	Anxiousness	Anxiousness	Negative outlook	Anxiousness
	Mistrustfulness	Suspiciousness	Mistrust	Separation insecurity
	Anger	Depressivity		
	Depressiveness	(Hostility)		
	Shame			
	Vulnerability			

Table A2   Continued

	FFiCD	PID-5 algorithm	Clark et al. scales	PID5BF+M
Detachment	Social detachment Emotional detachment Unassertiveness	Withdrawal Intimacy avoidance Restricted affectivity	Social detachment Emotional detachment	Withdrawal Intimacy avoidance Anhedonia
Dissociality	Lack of empathy Self-centredness Aggression	Callousness Grandiosity Manipulativeness Attention seeking Hostility	Low empathy Entitled superiority	Callousness Grandiosity Manipulativeness
Disinhibition	Irresponsibility Rashness Disorderliness Thrill seeking	Irresponsibility Impulsivity Distractibility Risk taking	Reckless impulsivity Distractibility	Irresponsibility Impulsivity Distractibility
Anankastia	Inflexibility Perfectionism Workaholism	Rigid perfectionism Perseveration	Hypercontrol Perfectionism	Rigidity Perfectionism Orderliness

Note. FFiCD = Five-Factor Inventory for ICD-11; PID-5 = Personality Inventory for DSM-5; PID5BF+M = Personality Inventory for DSM-5 and ICD-11 – Brief Form – Plus Modified.

Table A3 Five-Factor Inventory for ICD-11 with 20 facets and 47 nuances

Negative Affectivity	Detachment	Dissociality	Disinhibition	Anankastia
Anxiousness	**Emotional detachment**	**Aggression**	**Disorderliness**	**Inflexibility**
Evaluation apprehension	Joylessness	Passive aggression	Disorderliness	Dogmatism
Separation insecurity	Physical anhedonia	Physical aggression	Disorganised speech	Rigidity
Social anxiousness	Social anhedonia	Verbal aggression		Risk aversiveness
				Ruminative deliberation
Depression	**Social detachment**	**Lack of empathy**	**Irresponsibility**	**Perfectionism**
Interpersonal inadequacy	Coldness	Callousness	Impersistence	Fastidiousness
Pessimism	Social isolation	Exploitativeness	Distractibility	Punctiliousness
Suicidality		Manipulativeness	Ineptitude	
Worthlessness			Disobliged	
Emotional lability	**Unassertiveness**	**Self-centredness**	**Rashness**	**Workaholism**
Affective dysregulation		Arrogance	Rash behaviours	Doggedness
Rapidly shifting emotions		Entitlement	Rash thinking	Work preoccupation

Table A3   Continued

Negative Affectivity	Detachment	Dissociality	Disinhibition	Anankastia
		Selfishness		
		Vanity		
Shame			**Thrill seeking**	
Humiliation				
Self-consciousness				
Vulnerability				
Fragility				
Need for admiration				
Anger				
Annoyed				
Dysregulated anger				
Reactive anger				
Mistrustfulness				

Note. Bolded terms are facets, while others represent underlying nuances, all of which can be portrayed with the Five-Factor Inventory for ICD-11.

Appendix B
Translation From Traditional ICD-10 Types

It should not be forgotten that the diagnosis of Personality Disorder is rooted in a long and rich tradition of different types of Personality Disorders as we know them from ICD-10 and DSM-5. In order to maintain continuity with the knowledge and research based on these categories, some clinicians may find it practical and helpful to "translate" from the old types to the new classification. Therefore, here in Appendix B we will give the reader an overview of how traditional types of Personality Disorder can be understood in the new classification of severity and specification of trait domains. In particular, we will address Avoidant Personality Disorder and Narcissistic Personality Disorder, which may seem difficult to describe in ICD-11, as opposed to other types that are more straightforward (e.g., Anankastia and Anankastic Personality Disorder; Dissociality and Dissocial Personality Disorder).

Severity and Traditional Types

Traditionally, different types of Personality Disorder have been seen as expressions of how defense mechanisms and reality testing, among other things, function at different levels on a spectrum ranging from neurotic to psychotic functioning. Otto Kernberg (1967, 2019) has described this dimension as the organisational levels of personality functioning, which can be broadly equated to the severity of Personality Disorder (Caligor et al., 2018).

In a recent Danish study, clinicians were asked to characterise a total of 247 patients or clients by assessing their overall severity of personality dysfunction according to ICD-11 and indicating the ICD-10 Personality Disorder type(s) that best described them (Simon & Bach, 2022). As illustrated in Figure B1, a general pattern emerged from the responses. For example, there is a tendency for anankastic (i.e., obsessive-compulsive), dependent, and avoidant types to be ranked within Mild to Moderate Personality Disorder, while emotionally unstable (i.e., borderline), dissocial (i.e., antisocial), and paranoid are primarily ranked as Severe Personality Disorder.

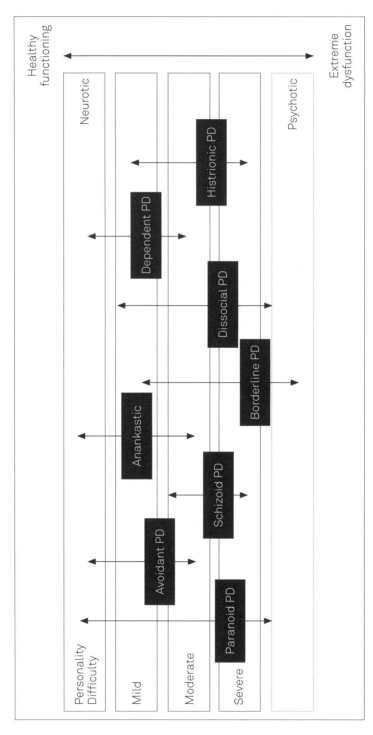

Figure B1 Types of Personality Disorder ranked by severity (inspired by Simon and Bach, 2022).

Trait Domains and Traditional Types

By acting as relatively homogeneous "building blocks" of personality pathology, trait domains help to illuminate and separate the more overlapping characteristics we know from the traditional categories of Personality Disorder. As a result, the "old" types often include different combinations of trait domains.

Obviously, Negative Affectivity plays a crucial role in several traditional types of Personality Disorder. Interpersonal aspects of Negative Affectivity (e.g., inferiority and dependency) are present in Dependent Personality Disorder (e.g., fear of separation from a supportive person) and Borderline Personality Disorder (e.g., frantic efforts to avoid abandonment or rejection). Similarly, anxious aspects of Negative Affectivity play a role in both Anankastic Personality Disorder (e.g., feelings of excessive doubt and caution) and Avoidant Personality Disorder (e.g., risk aversion due to a fear of feeling shame). Furthermore, we also see that the trait domains of Dissociality and Disinhibition are both involved in Dissocial Personality Disorder (e.g., very low tolerance for frustration and a low threshold for aggression and violence) and Borderline Personality Disorder (e.g., proneness to outbursts of anger or violence and inability to control the resulting behavioural explosions). Similarly, we see aspects of Dissociality in both Paranoid Personality Disorder (e.g., a combative and persistent sense of self-righteousness that does not match the actual situation) and Anankastic Personality Disorder (e.g., unreasonable insistence that others submit to one's way of doing things). In light of this, it is not surprising that there is a lot of overlap among the traditional Personality Disorder types.

It seems intuitively fitting to describe traditional types such as Anankastic Personality Disorder and Dissocial Personality Disorder in terms of trait domains. Thus, Dissociality captures the essence of Dissocial Personality Disorder. Similarly, Anankastic Personality Disorder can be directly described using the trait domain of Anankastia, while different variants of it can be portrayed based on combinations with other trait domains (see Chapter 6). Consistent with the restrictive personality style and behaviour associated with Anankastic Personality Disorder, the trait domain of Anankastia is also a particularly "clean" and "restricted" dimension, psychometrically speaking.

In contrast to the aforementioned types, Borderline Personality Disorder is the most heterogeneous and complex of all the types, which is best characterised using multiple trait domains. The mildest cases can be described solely by Negative Affectivity (e.g., emotional lability with low frustration tolerance), whereas more severe cases will typically include Negative Affectivity combined with Disinhibition (e.g., impulsivity and reckless behaviour), Dissociality (e.g., expectation of other's attention and anger when not granted), and sometimes even Detachment (e.g., limited capacity for enjoyment) and Anankastia (e.g., put extreme demands on themselves and others). This heterogeneity, with variation in severity and stylistic expressions, may explain some of the mixed and inconclusive research findings we encounter in studies on the treatment of Borderline Personality Disorder (Bohus et al., 2021; Johansen et al., 2004; Mulder & Tyrer, 2023; Sharp, 2018).

Table B1 provides a guide for translation between Personality Disorders in ICD-10 and trait domains in ICD-11, which is based on a review of nine scientific studies (Bach et al., 2018; Bach, Kerber et al., 2020; Fang et al., 2021; García et al., 2022; Kim et al., 2021; Lugo et al., 2019; Sellbom et al., 2020, 2023; Simon et al., 2023; Sorrel et al., 2022).

Table B1   Tentative translation from ICD-10 personality disorders to ICD-11 trait domains

	Negative Affectivity	Detachment	Dissociality	Disinhibition	Anankastia
Paranoid	+	+	+		
Schizoid		++			
Dissocial	−		++	++	
Borderline	++		+	++	
Histrionic	+	−	+	+	
Anankastic	+			−	++
Avoidant	++	++			+
Dependent	++			+[a]	
Narcissistic	+		++	+	+

Note. The symbols indicate when trait domains are very prominent (++) and prominent (+) while trait domains that typically occur in terms of a reversed score (−) can also be taken into account.
[a]Primarily applies to aspects of irresponsibility. Based on a review by Simon et al. (2023).

Avoidant Personality Disorder

Patients who would traditionally be diagnosed with Avoidant Personality Disorder can usually be classified as having a Mild, Moderate, or even Severe Personality Disorder, with mild to moderate severity being the most common. Their sense of self is characterised by inferiority and shame, which is driving their interpersonal struggles in terms of intense fear of criticism and rejection. Thus, their ability to understand others' perspectives is typically compromised by a distorted inference of others' perspectives as being negative. Their ability to work towards a goal is often compromised due to risk aversion, lack of confidence, and fear of being ashamed. Their relationships are characterised by avoidance, even intimate relationships, and their social and occupational roles are compromised due to social avoidance. Individuals with this pattern typically do not cause significant harm to others, but may cause some harm to themselves (e.g., a self-suppressive or self-defeating lifestyle).

In terms of Negative Affectivity, this pattern particularly involves anxiousness, shame, low self-esteem, and a tendency to be hyperreactive to perceived threats, criticism, or potential future problems. These patients' low self-esteem and lack of confidence manifest in the form of avoidance of situations and activities that are perceived to be too difficult (e.g., intellectually, physically, socially, interpersonally). In terms of Detachment, the anxious–avoidant pattern involves a social distance in the form of avoidance, lack of friendships, and avoidance of intimacy. Due to anxiousness and low self-esteem, such individuals either avoid social interactions altogether or endure them with extreme discomfort and/or use of safety behaviours. These patients either engage in little or no small talk, even if initiated by others (e.g., a shop assistant). They typically seek jobs that do not involve interaction with others, and they may turn down promotions or assignments if they involve more social interaction. The complete pattern of high Negative Affectivity and Detachment is generally consistent with the description of avoidant patients as being both fearful and emotionally inhibited (Fassbinder & Arntz, 2018; Simonsen et al., 2021). In addition, avoidant characteristics can also be elucidated by scales measuring facets and nuances of the trait domains in ICD-11 such as social anxiousness, evaluation apprehension, social isolation, shame, interpersonal inadequacy, risk aversiveness, worthlessness, and fragility (see Table A3 in Appendix A).

Narcissistic Personality Disorder

Individuals with a Narcissistic Personality Disorder may be characterised by features ranging from Mild to Severe Personality Disorder (Day et al., 2024). Their self-view can fluctuate between overly positive and inflated (e.g., almighty) to extraordinarily negative and deflated (e.g., powerless). Depending on the specific nature (i.e., grandiose or vulnerable) of the narcissistic disorder, such individuals may have difficulty recovering from even the slightest injury to their grandiose and vulnerable self-view. Thus, they may exhibit poor emotion regulation in the face of even minor threats to their self-esteem. Their self-centredness and lack of empathy can compromise the quality of their relationships, especially because other people's opinions do not really matter or because of interpersonal exploitation. They have few or no close mutual relationships, and existing relationships are often one-sided, where the narcissistic individual may appear highly dominant and unable to see the matter from multiple sides or from a more integrated understanding of the other person. For the same reason, a subset of these patients may be unable to maintain normal working relationships or cooperate with other people at all.

Narcissistic Personality Disorder is fundamentally characterised by the trait domain of Dissociality with an emphasis on self-centredness (Bach et al., 2018; Simon et al., 2023). This pattern involves the exploitation of others, underpinned by an entitled belief in deserving whatever one wants, which, according to such individuals, should be obvious to others. Such traits of narcissism can manifest in the expectation of others' admiration, attention-seeking behaviour, and anger or aggression when admiration and attention are not granted. These types of patients typically believe that their achievements are exceptional, that they have many admirable qualities, that they have or will achieve greatness, and that others should admire them. Many individuals with narcissistic features are also characterised by traits of Anankastia in the form of perfectionism, vanity, and stubbornness, which tend to sustain their competitiveness, inflated sense of self-esteem, and grandiose self-presentation (Fjermestad-Noll et al., 2020). Therefore, the combination of Dissociality and Anankastia can often indicate a narcissistic issue (Bach et al., 2018; Simon et al., 2023). Likewise, Negative Affectivity in the form of vulnerability, depressivity, anger, and shame can also be vulnerable manifestations of narcissism. Thus, the combination of Dissociality and Negative Affectivity can characterise individuals with vulnerable narcissism who easily feel dishonoured and continue to brood over what they perceive as insults from others (i.e., narcissistic injuries). Their low self-esteem issues can manifest as envy, and it can also be fuelled by shame over repeated failures and lack of success in their lives. Taken together, individual manifestations of narcissism can thus be captured by characteristic combinations of trait domains, with Dissociality serving as the main component. In addition, narcissistic traits can also be elucidated by scales measuring facets and nuances of the trait domains in ICD-11 such as entitlement, vanity, arrogance, selfishness, reactive anger, need for admiration, self-centredness, lack of empathy, perfectionism, and in the most vulnerable cases also shame, fragility, and evaluation apprehension (see Table A3 in Appendix A).

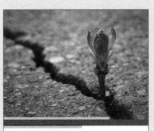

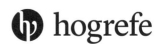

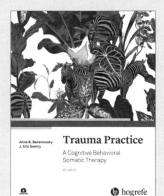
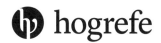

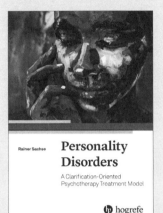
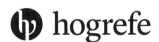